MEDICINE

POCKET LIBRARY OF SPIRITUAL WISDOM

Practical Applications

Also in this series:

RUDOLF STEINER

MEDICINE
An Introductory Reader

Compiled with an introduction, commentary and notes by Andrew Maendl, M.B., B.S. London

Sophia Books

All translations revised by Matthew Barton

Sophia Books
An imprint of Rudolf Steiner Press
Hillside House, The Square
Forest Row, RH18 5ES

www.rudolfsteinerpress.com

Published by Rudolf Steiner Press 2003

For earlier English publications of individual selections please
see pp. 218–19

The material by Rudolf Steiner was originally published in
German in various volumes of the 'GA' (*Rudolf Steiner
Gesamtausgabe* or Collected Works) by Rudolf Steiner Verlag,
Dornach. This authorized volume is published by permission of
the Rudolf Steiner Nachlassverwaltung, Dornach (for further
information see pp. 225–6)

This edition translated © Rudolf Steiner Press 2003

A catalogue record for this book is available from the British
Library

ISBN 1 85584 133 9

Cover by Andrew Morgan Design
Typeset by DP Photosetting, Aylesbury, Bucks.
Printed and bound in Great Britain by Cromwell Press Limited,
Trowbridge, Wilts.

Contents

Introduction

by Andrew Maendl, MD

This book presents some of Steiner's lectures and writings on medicine with a few explanatory comments. The essence of Steiner's approach is holistic, i.e. not confined to sense-perceptible physical phenomena, but encompassing the whole person of body, life-forces, soul and spirit, or, to use the terms Steiner used in his anthroposophy (wisdom of man), physical, etheric, astral and ego.

Steiner frequently refers to the fact that the modern scientific approach is insufficient on its own for gaining insight into deeper aspects of the human being. This selection from his writings and lectures — some of which were for doctors and others for a more general audience — starts by emphasizing intuition as an essential inner tool for really understanding what is at work in medicine. There follow chapters which describe the complexity of human supersensible 'bodies' above and beyond the physical. A holistic view is also presented of the opposite poles of cancer and inflammation, as well as case histories illumined through anthroposophical insight. This book gives a taste of the aims and practice of anthroposophical medicine, and of ways to pursue and implement it.

People have always asked themselves questions such as the following. Is our thinking just a secretion of our brain or is the brain in fact an instrument of our spirit? Are atoms and molecules the prime movers of physiology or are biochemical changes an expression of non-physical forces that work holistically? Is the world one big chance event or is there meaning in all creation and destiny? Are natural forces the only reality or are moral forces real too? Is death the end of existence or are near-death experiences a taste of another realm that we enter after death? Do we just appear out of nothing at birth or do we exist before this in a previous life?

Do we have to make do with suppositions in response to these questions or is it possible to really know the answers to some of them? Our spiritual values have increasingly been eroded by the march of reductionist science, affecting our attitudes and behaviour towards plants, animals and fellow human beings. This certainly gives rise to unease about the way civilization is going, despite the enormous boon of technological advance; yet we need more than a feeling of unease. A real knowledge is required of the deeper forces at work in the kingdoms of nature and the human being. Rudolf Steiner in his anthroposophy offers us ways to develop knowledge appropriate to our Western consciousness, without belittling or rejecting the real achievements of the modern mind.

First, though, an historical overview is helpful to understand how medicine developed. Let us look at medical practice in the pre-Christian mystery centres, where priests sought guidance from the spiritual world.

> ... In those olden times there was not so much experimenting as there is today. The sick person was brought into the temple and put into a kind of som- nambulistic condition by temple priests who were properly trained. This condition was increased to the level at which the sick person could describe the process of his illness. Then an opposite somnambulistic condi- tion was brought about and the temple priest was told the dream that contained the therapy. This was the manner of enquiry in the oldest mysteries; it led from disease to cure. And so it was that medical science was cultivated in olden times, by seeking knowledge of man through the human being himself.[1]

In such a pre-Christian mystery centre, the function of the priest was to seek guidance through communication with the gods. The impulse of the mystery centres dried up before Christian times, and after Christ's life on earth many human beings sought spiritual guidance through the Christian impulse instead of from these ancient mys- tery sources. In earlier times the spiritual forces working within nature were perceived and acknowledged. This was still the case at the time of the Celtic Christian Church. When this Church ceased to be active, nature came to be regarded as imbued with heathen powers. Knowledge of the way the spirit worked in nature was lost, and gradually we came to acquire our present abstract and reductionist view of natural forces.

After the Middle Ages Vesalius dissected corpses. While this led to greater anatomical awareness, it was also symptomatic of 'dead' knowledge about the body. Pathology was studied in the physical changes of organs, then tissues and cells, and more recently in the molecular biology of DNA. Thus the study of disease, which originated from communication with the gods in the mystery centres, has developed by slow contraction to a focus on minute, physical particles. More recently there has been a reverse swing towards holism. How can we retain the objectivity we have learnt from natural science, yet redirect it to encompass a much broader view of our place in the universe and interconnections with it? Steiner's work is imbued with this striving, as one can glean from the following excerpt:

> ... Our contemporary critics are certainly entitled to complain that our present observations are difficult to understand; yet the blackbird does not find them difficult—but easy and a matter of course. And this bird gives the most practical proof of its easy understanding. For the blackbird is not exactly an ascetic and therefore it occasionally devours poisonous spiders.[2] And when it begins to feel discomfort as a result—for such discomfort is soon considerable—and a henbane plant is near at hand, the blackbird makes a straight line for the henbane, knowing the appropriate remedy. And it

certainly is a remedy, for if there were no henbane available the blackbird could fall into convulsions and die in the most violent paroxysms. If the plant is near at hand, the bird is saved from a painful death by its own protective instinct which makes it pick and devour the remedy. This is the everyday event which furnishes us with an illustration.

The more remote example has substantial similarity with the case of the blackbird and henbane. Mankind must have developed certain protective and remedial instincts at a very primitive epoch, and these instincts must have supplied some of the content gathered in the Hippocratic school of medicine. Let us consider, in the light of the criticism referred to at the beginning of this chapter, the wisdom of the blackbird — or of other birds, who act in the same manner under similar circumstances. [...] The bird seeks help from the henbane. And why? Because in the very moment that the poison begins to work, this calls into activity the defensive and protective instinct; the instinctive awareness of injury passes over into the instinct of defence. And so in this phenomenon we have a very well-adapted development of what we ourselves do if a fly settles on our eyelid and we instantaneously close our eye and brush it off with our hand, by a simple reflex action. We may learn a very great deal from these instinctive actions of animals and plants. Their observation will help to cure us of another error: *the conviction that everything deserving the name of intelligence or reason has its seat in the skull only.*

Intelligence and reason hover everywhere, so to speak, for the bird's instinct for self-protection against injury illustrates intelligent behaviour. External reason and external intelligence are at work in such a case, while we human beings have simply the gift of sharing in this working of external forces. We share in it, but we do not contain it within ourselves. To say we do so is nonsense, but we participate in it.

The bird does not yet participate in it in such a way as to appropriate the instincts for protection against injury in a special portion of the body, namely, the brain. Birds' understanding operates more through their pulmonary system than ours — for mankind understands through the head system; and the bird's defensive instinct leads it to the henbane or *Hyoscyamus* [*niger*] through the pulmonary system, because the creature thinks less in its periphery than at the centre of its being. Mankind has detached the power of thought from lungs and the rhythmic system. Later on perhaps we may consider our human instruments of thought in more detail. But it is beyond question that we no longer think so centrally — that is, with heart, lungs and so forth, in unison with the cosmos, as birds still think. These are aptitudes that we must re-acquire. And if you ask what has expelled the last vestige of those instincts which link us to the whole of nature, the reply must be: the education we receive at school and university — for this, and everything related to it, is eminently suited to uproot man's interconnection with the totality of nature. Our education exerts a one-sided influence, promoting refined intellectuality on the one side, and refined sexuality on the other. The force which worked centrally in primeval mankind is driven apart in modern man towards these two polar opposites.

To find the way back to a right and sound understanding of the world it is necessary for our pursuit of science to become sound again [...]

Let us now turn to the possibility referred to yesterday of studying man in such a way that we get some hint of the therapeutic process. In archaic times this was a highly developed instinct. When primitive man found anything abnormal within himself he was at the same time led to the healing process. Modern mankind has lost these capacities, and therefore only very rarely reaches by intuition what ancient mankind found instinctively. But *that is the course of evolution: from instinct through intellectualism to intuition.*[3]

Thus we can gather that intuition is an essential approach for a medicine that wishes to work with the spiritual aspect of the human being, and a whole chapter will be devoted to this subject.

Who was Rudolf Steiner? Briefly, he was an initiate who developed understanding of the spiritual in man and nature in a way appropriate for our Western culture and form of consciousness. He underwent a scientific training which he said enabled him to reach much further into spiritual reality than if he had not had this. He produced a prodigious output of work: 28 books and about 6000 lectures.

Reading Steiner is not always easy. He himself says of his work *The Philosophy of Freedom* that it cannot be read as an ordinary book, but needs a great amount of inner thought and work. This can be said about much of his other work too. There is an enormous amount of information in Steiner's work. He was always most emphatic that what he says should *not* be accepted as blind belief but be checked and tested. Much of his work is not immediately and completely comprehensible at first, for he did not go out of his way to make his text easy, saying that the 'spiritual scientific' path of anthroposophy is nothing if not hard. One is therefore frequently thrown back on one's own resources, has to try to work out of one's own experience, do one's own research.

One exercise that interested readers may find helpful is just to read one of his lectures seven times. At first the text may seem difficult and dry. By the third reading it has become a full experience, by the seventh reading it seems like a familiar piece of music. Christopher Lindenau has devised a technique of sevenfold reading based on the following steps:[4]

1) just reading the text;
2) repeating it in one's own words;
3) how one reacts to it emotionally, what strikes one especially;
4) questions that arise from the text;

5) reading it *backwards* paragraph by paragraph to reveal the structure of the lecture;
6) meditating on it;
7) seeing what new experiences arise from all this work.

I have found this most helpful in practice.

Steiner stresses on many occasions that a true understanding of the human being cannot rely on schematic divisions into different 'parts'. While Steiner offers a conceptual basis for his view of man, which we will encounter in the following pages, he is also continually at pains to point out that this 'empty cupboard', which in itself remains abstract, needs to be filled with the experiential 'garments' of life itself and all its rich complexity.

> These things, however, become objectively living forms when we go into what is revealed in human life, in man's relations to the world, in what in any way is revealed by the world and what gives a certain definite content to the concepts which to begin with are limited to a preliminary plan [...] It is a great mistake if we believe we are doing something real in setting up a mere plan which is there, to start with, to provide us with the framework within which our observations may be contained.[5]

Because Steiner, as a true scientist, was always more interested in life itself than in theories about it, some statements he makes in the following pages may seem to contradict each other on occasion. Such apparent contradictions only occur, however, when they remain abstract, divorced from specific, real situations and contexts. His statements often need to be raised to the sphere of experience before they make sense, and then apparent contradictions are usually reconciled. Sometimes one may have to live with certain statements for years before they suddenly reveal their secrets in a flash. Steiner's work, as we have seen, is not always easily accessible, but the struggle to comprehend some of the most difficult passages is frequently repaid by illuminating and original insights.

There is a great deal of dissatisfaction in medicine today, and this may partly be due to the prevailing superficial view of the human being as a creature composed more or less entirely of complex biochemistry. Deep down most doctors sense that there is a great deal more to human nature. Steiner has given us a path, albeit a difficult one, for discovering deeper aspects of the human being, upon which a true art of healing can be based.

1. Understanding Man's True Nature as a Basis for Medical Practice

The following is the first chapter of the book Fundamentals of Therapy,[1] *which was Steiner's last book. It is unusual in that he wrote it together with another person, Dr Ita Wegman, a leading doctor in the anthroposophical movement with whom he had a close connection. This chapter presents a very full and succinct introduction to anthroposophical medicine. In particular it stresses the importance of the way we regard or understand the human being, and the effect this can have – for good or ill – on our capacities to heal. Steiner also outlines ways to develop a new power of concentrated thinking that can lead to new medical insights. He says that each of the three modes of perception that we can develop beyond our ordinary faculties is intimately related to three different constituent aspects of the human being (living processes, soul life and the innermost spiritual core) and a tool for understanding these. Steiner and Wegman here elaborate on the path of cognition pursued by spiritual science, and describe the complex interaction of the ego or 'I' and the astral, etheric and physical bodies in health and illness.[2]*

This small book presents new approaches in medical knowledge and skills [...] It is not a matter of being in opposition to the school of medicine that is working with the accepted scientific methods of the present time. We fully acknowledge its principles. And in our view, the approach we present should only be used by those who are fully able and entitled to practise medicine according to those principles.

We do, however, add further insights to such knowledge of the human being as is now available through accepted scientific methods. These are gained by different methods, and we therefore feel compelled to work for an extension of clinical medicine based on these *wider* insights into the nature of the world and the human being.

Basically, those who follow established medical practice cannot object to what we are presenting because we do not go against that practice. The only people who can refuse to accept our attempt without further ado are those who not only demand that we accept their system of knowledge but also insist that no insights may be presented that go beyond their system.

Extended insight into the nature of the world and the human being is in our view offered in anthroposophy, an approach established by Rudolf Steiner. To our understanding of the *physical* human being, which can only be gained by the methods of natural science,[3] it adds understanding of the *non-physical* or *spiritual* human being. Anthroposophy does not involve progressing from insight into the physical to insight into the spiritual aspect by merely thinking about it. This would only produce more or less well thought-out hypotheses, with no one able to prove that they are in accord with reality.

Before anything is said in anthroposophy about the spiritual aspect, methods are developed that entitle one to make such statements. To get some idea of these methods, readers are asked to consider the following. All findings made in established modern science are essentially based on impressions gained through the human senses. Human beings may extend their ability to perceive what the senses can provide by means of experiments or through observations made using instruments, but this adds nothing *essentially* new to knowledge gained in that world in which human beings live through their senses.

Thinking, in so far as it is applied to investigating the physical world, also does not add anything to the evidence of our senses. In thinking we combine or analyse sensory impressions to arrive at laws (of nature); those who investigate the world of the senses must, however, say to themselves: the thinking which thus arises in me does not add anything real to the reality of the world perceived by the senses.

This will change as soon as human beings do not limit themselves to the level and type of thinking that they initially develop through life, upbringing and education. We can strengthen our thinking and increase its power. We can focus the mind on simple, limited thoughts and then, excluding all other thoughts, concentrate the whole power of soul on such ideas. A muscle gains in strength if tensed repeatedly, the forces exerted always focused in the same direction. Inner powers of soul are strengthened in the sphere that normally governs thinking by practising exercises in this concentrated way. It has to be emphasized that the exercises must be based on simple, limited thoughts, for the soul should not be exposed to influences that are half or even fully unconscious during those exercises. [For full details and directions on how to practise such exercises, see Rudolf Steiner's *How to Know Higher Worlds, Occult Science* and other anthroposophical writings listed under Further Reading.]

The most obvious objection to this is that if the whole power of soul is directed to a specific thought, focusing on it completely, all kinds of autosuggestion and the like may arise, and one simply begins to imagine things. Anthroposophy however also teaches how the exercises should be practised in a way that renders such objection null and void. In doing these exercises one proceeds in full presence of mind just as one does in solving a problem in arithmetic or geometry. The mind cannot lapse into unconscious spheres when solving such problems, nor can it do so if the directions given in anthroposophy are carefully followed.

Doing these exercises strengthens the *powers of thought* to a previously undreamt-of degree. We feel powers of thought active in us like a new content in the essence of our being. And as our own being is given new content, the world, too, is perceived to have a content of which we may have had a vague idea before but which we have not known from experience. Considering our ordinary thinking in moments of self-observation, we find our thoughts to be shadow-like and pale compared to impressions gained through the senses.

Perceptions gained through enhanced powers of thinking are far from pale and shadowy; they are full of content, utterly real images; their reality is much more intense than is found in the content of our sensory impressions. A new world opens up for human beings when they have extended their powers of perception in the way indicated.

As people learn to have perceptions in this world of thought where before they were only able to have perceptions in the world of the senses, they realize that all the laws of nature they knew before apply *only* in the physical world; and that the nature of the world they have now entered is such that its laws are different, indeed the opposite of those in the physical world. In this world, the law of the earth's force of attraction does not apply, but rather the opposite, for a force presents itself that does not act outwards from the centre of the earth but the other way round, from the periphery of the universe to the centre of the earth. And the same holds true for the other forces of the physical world.

In anthroposophy, the ability to perceive this world, gained through exercises, is called the power of imaginative perception[4] — imaginative not because one is dealing with 'figments of the imagination' but because the contents of the conscious mind are not thought shadows but images. Sensory perception gives direct experience of being in a real world, and so does the inner activity of gaining imaginative knowledge. The world to which this perception relates is called the etheric world in anthroposophy. This is not the hypothetical ether of modern physics, but something truly perceived in the spirit. The name is used because it relates to earlier, instinctive ideas of this world. Compared to the clear perceptions now possible such antiquated ideas no longer have validity; but we have to give names to things if we wish to refer to them.

Within this ether world it is possible to perceive an etheric bodily nature that exists in addition to the human being's physical bodily nature. Our etheric bodily nature is something that in essence exists also in the plant world. Plants have an ether body. The laws of physics, as such, actually apply only in the world of lifeless minerals.

The plant world is possible on earth because there are substances in the earth-sphere that are not limited to the laws of physics but may leave all physical laws behind and adopt laws that go in the opposite direction. The laws of physics act as though streaming out from the earth; etheric laws act as though streaming into the earth from all directions of the universe. We can only understand the developing plant world if we see how in it earthly physical principles interact with etheric and cosmic principles.

And that is how it is with regard to the human etheric body. Because of it, something happens in the human being that is not a continuation of forces of the physical body acting according to their own laws, but happens because physical substances rid themselves of their physical forces as soon as they stream into the etheric realm.

At the beginning of a human life on earth — most clearly so during the embryonic period — the forces of the etheric body act as powers of synthesis and growth. As life progresses, a part of these forces becomes emancipated from activity in synthesis and growth and is transformed into powers of thought — the very powers that create the shadowy thought world we have in our ordinary consciousness.

It is of the greatest importance to know that ordinary human powers of thought are refined powers of synthesis and growth. A spiritual principle reveals itself in the synthesis and growth of the human organism. And as life progresses this principle emerges as the spiritual power of thought. And this power of thought is only one part of the power of human synthesis and growth that is at work in the etheric. The other part remains faithful to the function it had at the beginning of human life. Human beings continue to develop when synthesis and growth have reached an advanced stage, that is, to some degree a conclusion; and it is because of this that the non-physical, spiritual etheric which is alive and actively at work in the organism is able to become power of thought in later life.

The power to change and be changed thus presents itself to imaginative perception in one aspect as being etheric and spiritual, and in its other aspect as the soul content of thinking.

If we consider the material nature of earthly substances

and follow how etheric forces work on them, we have to say that wherever material substances enter into this creative process, they develop an essential nature that estranges them from physical nature. Becoming estranged, they enter into a world where the spiritual principle meets them and transforms them so that they assume its own nature.

To rise to the living, etheric nature of the human being in the way described here is something utterly different from the unscientific insistence on a 'vital force' that was commonly used in the attempt to explain living bodies up to the middle of the nineteenth century. Here it is a matter of directly perceiving—in mind and spirit—an essential principle that exists in humans and all other life forms just as the physical body does. To gain this perception we do not continue the ordinary way of thinking in some vague fashion, nor do we make up another world using our powers of fantasy. Instead, human perceptiveness is extended in a highly specific way, and this then also leads to experience of a wider world.[5]

The exercises that lead to such higher perception may be taken further. Having made an extra effort to concentrate on specific thoughts, it is also possible to make a further effort to suppress these imaginations (images of a spiritual, etheric reality) that have been achieved. The resulting state is a completely empty conscious mind. One is merely awake, and this waking state initially has no content.[6] This waking state without content does not continue, however. Having been emptied of all physical and all image-like etheric impressions, it fills with a content that streams to it from a real world of the spirit, just as impressions we gain of the physical world stream towards the physical senses.

Through imaginative perception we get to know a second aspect of our human nature; when the empty conscious mind fills with spiritual content as described we get to know a third aspect. In anthroposophy, perceptive insight arrived at in this way is said to come through Inspiration. [...] The world to which we gain access through Inspiration is called the astral world in anthroposophy. Speaking of an etheric world we refer to the influences that take effect from the periphery, the cosmos, and radiate in towards the earth. Speaking of an astral world, however, we progress, in accordance with what the inspired conscious mind observes, from influences coming towards us from the periphery to specific spirit entities revealed within those influences, just as the physical substances of the earth reveal their nature in the forces emanating from the earth. In the astral world we speak of distinct spirit entities acting from the far distances of the universe just as we speak of stars and constellations when we use our senses to look at the night sky. Hence the term 'astral world'.[7] In this astral world human beings have the third aspect of their essential nature: the astral body.

Earthly substantiality must also stream into this astral body. In the process it becomes further estranged from its physical nature. Human beings thus have their ether body in common with the plant world and their astral body with the animal world.[8]

The essentially human element that raises humanity above the animal world is perceived and becomes known through a form of perceptive insight that is still higher than Inspiration. This is called 'Intuition' in anthroposophy. In Inspiration a world of spiritual entities reveals itself. In Intuition the relationship of the perceiving human being to this world becomes a still closer one. Something purely spiritual is brought to conscious awareness, and this conscious awareness immediately shows that it has nothing to do with experience gained through our physical senses and bodily nature. We thus enter into a life where we are human spirit among other spiritual entities. In Inspiration the spiritual entities of the world *reveal* themselves; through Intuition, on the other hand, we *live with* those spirits.

We thus come to recognize the fourth aspect of essential human nature, the 'I' itself. Again, we become aware that in making itself part of the essence and active working of the 'I', earthly substantiality becomes even further estranged from its physical nature. The essential nature this substantiality assumes as 'I'-organization is initially the form in which earthly matter is most estranged from the physical nature it has on earth.[9]

The 'astral body' and 'I' we thus encounter are not tied to the physical body in the human organization in the way that the etheric or life body is. Inspiration and Intuition show that 'astral body' and 'I' separate from the physical and etheric bodies during sleep, and that complete inter-penetration of the four aspects of human nature to create an integral human entity exists only in the waking state.

In sleep, the physical and etheric human body remain in the physical and etheric world. They are not, however, in the position in which the physical and etheric body of a plant are. They retain the after-effects of the astral and 'I' principles. And the moment they no longer retain these after-effects the individual must wake up. A human physical body must never be left merely to physical influences, nor a human ether body merely to etheric influences, for then they would disintegrate.[10]

Inspiration and Intuition also show something else, however. Physical substantiality undergoes further development of its essential nature when it is raised to life and active work in the etheric. And this *life* depends on the organic, physical body being drawn away from earthly nature and built up by the universe that lies beyond the earth. Such synthesis and development only results in *life*, however, and not in *conscious awareness* nor in *self-awareness*. The astral body needs to build its organization within the physical and etheric organization; the 'I' needs to do the same with regard to the 'I' organization. Yet this *building-up process* does not lead to conscious development of an inner life of soul. For this to happen, synthesis and organic development has to be countered by *destruction*. The astral body builds its organs, then breaks them down again by letting the activity of feeling develop in the soul's inner awareness; the 'I' evolves its 'I' organization, then breaks it down again as will activity takes effect in self-awareness.

The spirit does *not* develop on the basis of *constructive* but of *destructive* activity of matter in the essential human being. If spirit is to be active in man, matter must withdraw from this activity.

Even the development of thinking activity within the etheric body is not based on a continuation of etheric nature but on its destruction. *Conscious* thinking does *not* take place in processes of synthesis and growth, but in processes of breakdown and withering, dying, which are continually integrated into the etheric process.

In conscious thinking, thoughts are freed from the physical synthesizing process and as soul configurations become living human experiences.

If we consider the human being on the basis of this approach to human nature, we realize that it is only possible to get full insight into both the human being as a whole and into an individual organ if we know how the physical body, the etheric body, the astral body and the 'I' are active in them. In some organs the 'I' is predominantly active; in others the 'I' shows little activity, and physical organization predominates.

We can only fully understand the healthy human being if we know how the higher aspects of human nature take hold of earthly substance and compel it to serve them, and if we also realize that earthly substance changes when raised into the sphere of activity of the higher aspects of human nature. In the same way we can only understand the sick human being if we realize the situation that arises for the organism as a whole, for an organ or a sequence of organs, if the mode of action of the higher principles becomes irregular. And we shall only be able to think of medicines when we develop knowledge of how an earthly substance or earthly process relates to the etheric, to the astral, to the 'I'. Only then will it be possible to introduce an earthly substance into the human organism or to treat the organism with an earthly activity to such effect that the higher aspects of the human being are able to develop unhindered or, of course, that earthly substantiality gains the support it needs from what has been added to it, so it may go in a direction where it becomes the foundation for the work of the spirit on earth.

Man is what he is through physical body, ether body, soul (astral body) and 'I' (spirit). In health human beings must be considered in terms of these aspects, in sickness perceived in terms of the balance between them being upset; for health, it is necessary to find medicines that will restore the upset balance. An approach to medicine based on these foundations is outlined in this book.

2. The Science of Knowing

As we have seen, Steiner's insights involve intensification of thinking from abstract greyness to intense experience, enabling one to gain perception of higher spiritual worlds. This sort of spiritual development requires great application and discipline. Higher levels of Intuition are achieved by very few people, though all of us have such faculties in incipient and often more unconscious form. Even if we cannot follow Steiner into the more rarefied areas where his perceptions and investigations lead him, with good will and healthy common sense, and by continually relating his insights to life in general and medical practice in particular, we can gain useful tools for enhancing our own understanding. When studying Steiner, and trying to put his insights to practical use in medicine, mere suspension of disbelief is not enough, and we are likely to face some of the following questions:

1) *How can we actually experience the functioning of the supersensible bodies he describes?*
2) *How can we experience the way the various remedies work on these supersensible bodies?*
3) *How can we transform the findings of modern science into a holistic experience?*

Is there a method with which we can tackle these questions? In the previous chapter Steiner tells us to work on the book How to

Know Higher Worlds. *This is a long arduous task, however, and meanwhile we have patients to attend to! Steiner recognized this difficulty and suggests in what follows that the very original, intuitive method Goethe developed in his scientific investigations is one we can usefully take up, without needing to develop immediate supersensible perception. This method begins to enable us to see specific instances (of illness for instance) as particular manifestations, different in each individual, of archetypal processes. Steiner is also at pains to point out the radical difference needed in our approach to organic life as opposed to inorganic phenomena. While one may find it difficult to penetrate all that is said here about the difference between natural law (inorganic) and* typus *(organic life), the important thing to draw from it is that in organic life cause and effect exist in a quite different mode, one we can only approach through developing an inner, imaginative and intuitive path of knowledge. To do so, according to Steiner, also involves 'a more intense activity of our spirit'. In other words we have to work in a more concentrated, inner way to grasp an archetype* (typus) *than a natural law, and, besides drawing on the intellect as we do in ordinary science, have to activate our feeling and will. Intellectual thinking separates us from the world, whereas if we suspend judgement for a time and just 'live with' the object under investigation, we unite with the phenomenon itself in a much deeper way. Thinking is not excluded from this process, but arises out of it. Steiner makes a rather unusual distinction at the end of this section between 'intellect' and 'reason'. The first he sees as separating the world into isolated concepts, the second as the unifying force which always posits a whole and seeks to link and connect.*

Outline of an epistemology implicit in Goethe's world view

A serious error has been committed [in modern science] in believing that the methods of inorganic science should simply be taken over into the realm of living organisms. It was considered that this method was the only scientific one, and that the study of organic life could only be truly scientific if it adhered to the same laws that underlie *physics* for example. The possibility was forgotten, however, that perhaps the concept of what is scientific is much broader than an explanation of the world according to the laws of the physical world. Even today people have not yet penetrated through to this knowledge. Instead of investigating what it is that makes the approach of the inorganic sciences scientific, and of then seeking a method that can be applied to the world of living things while adhering to the requirements that result from this investigation, scientists simply declared that the laws gained in this lower level of existence should be universally applied.

Above all, however, one should investigate what the basis is for any scientific thinking. [...] We saw already that inorganic laws are not the sole ones in existence but are only a special instance of all possible lawfulness in general. The method of physics is simply one *particular* case of a general scientific method of investigation [...] If this method is extended into the organic, one obliterates the specific nature of the organic. Instead of investigating the organic in accordance with its actual nature, one forces upon it a lawfulness alien to it [...]

All this comes from the erroneous view that the method of science is extraneous to its objects of study, that it is not determined by these objects or phenomena themselves but rather by *our* own nature. It is believed that one must think in a particular way about objects, that one must indeed think about *all* objects — throughout the entire universe — in the same way. Investigations are undertaken that are supposed to show that, due to the nature of our mind, we can think only deductively.

In doing so, however, one overlooks the fact that the objects or phenomena themselves may not tolerate the way of looking at them that we want to apply.

A look at the views of Haeckel, who is certainly the most significant of modern scientific theoreticians, shows us that the objection we are making to the organic natural science of our day is entirely justified, namely, that it does not carry over into organic nature the principle of scientific contemplation in the absolute sense, but only the principle of inorganic nature.

When he demands of all scientific striving that 'the *causal* interconnections of phenomena become recognized everywhere', when he says that 'if *psychological mechanisms* were not so infinitely complex, if we were also able to have a complete overview of the historical development of psychological functions, we would then be able to bring them all into a mathematical soul formula', then one can see clearly from this what he wants: *to treat the whole world according to the stereotype of the method of the physical sciences.*

This demand, however, does not underlie Darwinism in its original form but only in its present-day interpretation. We have seen that to explain a process in inorganic nature means to show its *lawful emergence* out of other sense-perceptible realities, to trace it back to objects that, like *itself*, belong to the sense world. But how does modern organic science employ the principles of *adaptation* and the *survival of the fittest* (both of which we certainly do not doubt are the expression of facts)? It is believed that one can trace the character of a particular species directly back to the outer conditions in which it lived, in somewhat the same way as the heating of an object is traced back to the rays of the sun falling upon it. One forgets completely that one can never show a species' character, with all its qualities, to be the result of these conditions. The conditions may have a determining influence, but they are not a *creating* cause. We can definitely say that under the influence of certain circumstances a species had to evolve in such a way that one or another organ became particularly developed; what is there as content, however, the specifically organic, cannot be derived from outer conditions. Let us say that an organic entity has the essential characteristics *abc*; then, under the influence of certain outer conditions, it has evolved. Through this, its characteristics have taken on the particular form *a′ b′ c′*. When we take these influences into account we will then understand that *a* has evolved into the form of *a′*, *b* into *b′*, *c* into c'. But the specific nature of a, b, and c can never arise as the outcome of external conditions.

One must, above all, focus one's thinking on asking from what we derive the content of that general 'something' of which we consider the individual organic entity to be a specialized case? We know very well that specialization comes from external influences. But we must trace the specialized shape itself back to an inner principle. We gain enlightenment as to why just this particular form has evolved when we study a creature's environment. But this particular form is, after all, something in and of itself; we see that it possesses certain inherent characteristics. We see what is essential. A content, configured in itself, confronts the outer phenomenal world, and this content provides us with what we need in tracing those characteristics back to their source. In inorganic nature we perceive a fact and see, in order to explain it, a second, a third fact and so on; and the result is that the first fact appears to us to be the necessary consequence of the other ones. In the organic world this is not so. There, in addition to the facts, we need yet another factor. We must see the influence of outer circumstances as confronted by something that does not passively allow itself to be determined by them but rather determines itself, actively, out of itself, under the influence of the outer circumstances.

But what is that basic factor? It can, after all, be nothing other than what manifests in the *general form* of a creature. A specific organism always manifests in particular, defined ways. The basic factor we are seeing is therefore to be found in the general characteristics of a particular organism: a *general image of the organism*, which comprises within itself all the particular forms of organisms.

Following Goethe's example, let us call this general organism *typus*. Whatever the word *typus* might mean etymologically, we are using it in this Goethean sense and never mean anything else by it than what we have indicated. This *typus* is not developed in all its completeness in any single organism. Only our thinking, in accordance with reason, is able to grasp it, by drawing it forth, as a general image, from phenomena. The *typus* is thus the underlying idea of the organism: the animal quality in the animal, the general plant (Goethe called it the *Urpflanze* or archetypal plant) in the specific one.

One should not picture this *typus* as anything rigid. It has nothing at all to do with what Agassiz, Darwin's most significant opponent, called 'an incarnate creative thought of God'. The *typus* is something altogether fluid, from which all the particular species and genera, which one can regard as subtypes or specialized types, can be derived. The *typus* does not preclude the theory of evolution. It does not contradict the *fact* that organic forms evolve out of one another. It is only reason's protest against the view that organic development consists purely in sequential, factual (sense-perceptible) forms. It is what underlies this whole development. It is what establishes interconnections in all this endless manifoldness. It is the inner aspect of what we experience as the outer forms of living things. *Darwinian theory presupposes the typus.*

The *typus* is the true archetypal organism [...] either archetypal plant or archetypal animal. It cannot be any single, sense-perceptible, actual living being. What Haeckel or other naturalists regard as the archetypal form is already a particular shape; it is, in fact, the simplest shape of the *typus*. The fact that in time the *typus* arises in its simplest form first does not require the forms evolving later to be the result of those preceding them in time. *All* forms result as a *consequence of the typus*; the first as well as the last are manifestations of it. We must take it as the basis of a true organic science and not simply undertake to derive the individual animal and plant species out of one another. The *typus* runs like a red thread through all the developmental stages of the organic world. We must hold onto it and then *with it* travel through this great realm of many forms. Then this realm will become understandable to us. Otherwise it falls apart for us, just as the rest of the world of experience does, into an unconnected mass of particulars. In fact, even when we believe that we are leading what is later more complicated, more compound, back to a *previous* simpler form, and that in the latter we have something original, even then we are deceiving ourselves, for we have only derived a specific form from a specific form.

Friedrich Theodor Vischer once said of Darwinian theory that it necessitates a revision of our concept of time. We have now arrived at a point that makes evident to us in what sense such a revision would have to occur. It would have to show that deriving something later out of something earlier is no explanation, that what is first in time is not first in principle. All deriving has to do with principles, and at best it could be shown which factors were at work such that one species of beings evolved *before* another one *in time*.

The *typus* plays the same role in the organic world as natural law does in the inorganic. Just as natural law provides us with the possibility of recognizing each individual phenomenon as a part of one great whole, so the *typus* enables us to regard the individual organism as a particular instance of the archetypal form.

We have already indicated that the *typus* is not a complete, frozen conceptual form, but that it is fluid, that it can assume the most manifold configurations. The number of these configurations is infinite, because what makes the archetypal form into a single particular form has no significance for the archetypal form itself. It is exactly the same as the way one law of nature governs infinitely many individual phenomena, because the specific conditions that arise in an individual case have nothing to do with the underlying law as such.

Nevertheless, we have to do here with something essentially different than in inorganic nature. There it is a matter of showing that a particular sense-perceptible fact can occur in this and in no other way, because this or that *natural law* exists. In the inorganic world fact and the law confront each other as two separate factors, and absolutely no further mental work is necessary except, when we become aware of a fact, to remember the law that applies.

This is different in the case of a living being and its manifestations. Here it is a matter of developing, out of the *typus* that we need to grasp, the individual form arising in our experience. We must carry out a mental process of an essentially different kind. We may not simply contrast the *typus* as something finished, in the way the natural law is, with the individual phenomenon.

The fact that every object, if it is not prevented by incidental circumstances, falls to the earth in such a way that the distances covered in successive intervals of time are in the ratio 1:3:5:7, etc., is a definite *law* that is fixed once and for all. It is an *archetypal phenomenon* that occurs when two masses (the earth and an object upon it) enter into interrelationship. If now a specific case enters the field of our observation to which this law is applicable, we then need only look at the facts observable to our senses in the context with which the law provides us, and we will find this law to be confirmed. We lead the individual case back to the law. This natural law expresses the connection of the facts that are separated in the sense world; but it continues to exist as such independently of the individual phenomenon. With the *typus* we must *develop* the particular case we find before us *out* of the archetypal form. We may not contrast the *typus* with the individual form in order to see how it governs the latter; we must allow the individual form to *arise from the typus*. A law governs the phenomenon as something standing over it, whereas the *typus* flows into an individual living being, and identifies itself with it.

If an organic science wants to be a science in the sense that mechanics or physics is, it must therefore know the *typus* to be the most general form and must then show it also in diverse, ideal, separate shapes. Mechanics is indeed also a compilation of diverse natural laws where the real determinants are altogether hypothetically assumed. It must be no different in organic science. Here also one would have to assume hypothetically determined forms in which the *typus* develops itself if one wanted to have a rational science. One would then have to show how these hypothetical configurations can always be brought to a definite form that exists for our observation.

Just as in the inorganic we lead a phenomenon back to a law, so here we *develop* a specific form out of the archetypal form. Organic science does not come about by outwardly juxtaposing the general and the particular, but rather by developing one form out of the other.

Just as mechanics is a system of natural laws, so organic science is meant to be a series of developmental forms of the *typus*. It is just that in mechanics we must bring the individual laws together and order them into a whole, whereas here we must allow the individual forms to go forth from one another in a living way.

It is possible to make an objection here. If the *typical* form (*typus*) is something altogether fluid, how is it at all possible to set up a chain of sequential, particular types as the content of an organic science? One can very well picture to oneself that, in every particular case one observes, one recognizes a specific form of the *typus*, but one cannot, after all, for the purposes of science, merely collect such real, observed cases.

One can do something else, however. One can let the *typus* run through its series of possibilities and then always (hypothetically) hold fast to this or that form. In this way one gains a series of forms, derived in thought from the *typus*, as the content of a *rational organic science*.

An organic science is possible which, like mechanics, is science in altogether the strictest sense. It is just that the method is a different one. The method of mechanics is to prove things. Every proof is based upon a certain principle. There always exists a particular presupposition (i.e. conditions are posited that can potentially be experienced in reality), and it is then determined what happens when these presuppositions occur. We then understand the individual phenomenon by applying the underlying law. We think about it like this: under these conditions, a phenomenon occurs; the conditions are there, so the phenomenon *must* occur. This is our thought process when we approach an event in the inorganic world in order to explain it. This is the method that proves things. It is scientific because it completely permeates a phenomenon with a concept, so that perception and thinking coincide.

But we can do nothing with this method of proving things in organic science. The *typus*, in fact, does not cause particular phenomena to occur under certain conditions; it determines nothing about a relationship between conditions that are alien to each other, that confront each other externally. It determines only the lawfulness of its own conditions and aspects. It does not point, like a natural law, beyond itself. Particular organic forms can therefore be developed only out of the general *typus* form, and the organic beings that arise in experience must coincide with one such derived form of the *typus*. The developmental method must here take the place of the proving one. One establishes here not that outer conditions affect each other in a certain way and thereby have a definite result, but rather that under definite outer circumstances a particular form has developed out of the *typus*. This is the far-reaching difference between inorganic and organic science. This difference underlies no investigative approach as consistently as the Goethean one. No one has recognized better than Goethe that an organic science, without recourse to opaque mysticism, without teleology, without assuming special creative powers, must be possible. But neither has anyone more vigorously rejected the unwarranted expectation of being able to accomplish anything in this realm by applying the methods of inorganic science.

The *typus*, as we have seen, is a fuller scientific form than the archetypal phenomenon in inorganic science. It also presupposes a more intensive mental activity on our part than the archetypal phenomenon does. As we reflect upon the things of inorganic nature, sense perception supplies us with the content. Our sense organization already supplies us with what in the organic realm we receive only through our mind and spirit. In order to perceive sweet, sour, warmth, cold, light, colour, etc., one need only have healthy senses. [...] In the *typus*, however, content and form are closely bound to each other. Therefore the *typus* does not in fact determine content purely in terms of form in the way a law does, but rather permeates the content in a living way, from within outwards, as its own. Our thinking mind is confronted with the task of participating productively in the creation of the content alongside the element of form.

The kind of thinking in which content appears in direct, living connection with the form element [*rather than as an external causal factor*] has always been called '*intuitive*'.

Intuition appears repeatedly as a scientific principle. The English philosopher Reid calls it an intuition when, out of our perception of outer phenomena (sense impressions), we acquire at the same time a conviction that they really *exist*. Jacobi thought that in our feeling of God we are given not only this feeling itself but at the same time the proof that God *is*. This judgement is also called intuitive. What is characteristic of intuition, as one can see, is always that more is given in the content than this content itself; one experiences a mental characterization *without proof*, merely through direct conviction. One believes it to be unnecessary to prove one's ideas and characterizations ('real existence' etc.) about the content of perception; in fact, one possesses them in undivided unity with the content.

It is really the same thing with the *typus*. It can offer no means of proof but can merely provide the possibility of developing every particular form out of itself. Our mind and spirit, consequently, must work much more intensively in grasping the *typus* than in grasping a natural law. It must produce content along with form. It must take upon itself an activity that the senses carry out in inorganic science and that we can call beholding. But at this higher level the spirit itself must be able to behold inwardly. Our power of judgement must be a *beholding in thought*, and *a thinking beheld*. We have to do here, as was expounded for the first time by Goethe, with a power to judge in beholding.[1] Goethe thereby revealed as a necessary form of human apprehension what Kant wanted to prove was something inaccessible to the human being, due to the innate limitations of his nature.

Just as in organic nature the *typus* takes the place of natural law, so in ourselves intuition takes the place of an evidence-based power of judgement. [...] People have often treated intuition in a very scornful way in science. It was regarded as a defect of Goethe's mind that he wanted to attain scientific truths through intuition. What is attained in an intuitive way is, in fact, considered by many to be quite important when it is a matter of a scientific *discovery*. There, one says, an *inspiration* often leads further than methodically trained thinking. One frequently calls it intuition, in fact, when someone by chance has hit upon something right, whose truth the researcher must first convince himself of by roundabout means. But it is always denied that intuition itself could be a principle of science. What occurs to intuition must afterwards first be proved — so it is thought — if it is to have any scientific value.

Thus people also considered Goethe's scientific achievements to be brilliant inspirations that only afterwards received credibility through strict science.

But for organic science, intuition is indeed the right method. It follows quite clearly from our considerations, we think, that Goethe's spirit found the right path in the organic realm precisely because it was intuitively predisposed. The method appropriate to the organic realm coincided with the constitution of his spirit. Because of this, the extent to which this method differs from that of inorganic science became increasingly clear to him. The one became clear to him through the other. He was therefore also able to sketch the nature of inorganic matter in clear strokes.

The belittling way in which intuition is treated is due in no small measure to the fact that one believes the same degree of credibility cannot be attributed to its achievements as to those of proof-based sciences. One often calls *knowing* only that which has been proved, and everything else *faith*.

One must bear in mind that intuition means something completely different within our scientific direction — which is convinced that in thinking we grasp the core of the world in its essential being — than in that direction which shifts this core into a beyond we cannot investigate. A person who sees in the world lying before us — in so far as we either experience it or penetrate it with our thinking—nothing more than a reflection (an image of some other-worldly, unknown, active principle that remains hidden behind this shell not only to one's first glance but also to all scientific investigation) can certainly regard the evidence-based method as nothing but a sub-stitute for the insight we lack into the *essential being* of things. Since he does not advance further to the view that a thought-connection comes about directly through the essential content given in thought, i.e., through the thing itself, he believes himself able to support this thought-connection only through the fact that it is in harmony with several basic convictions (axioms) so simple that they are neither susceptible to proof nor in need thereof. If such a person is then presented with a scientific statement without proof, a statement, indeed, that by its very nature excludes the method based on proof, then it seems to him to be externally imposed. A truth approaches him without his knowing what the basis of its validity is. He believes he has no knowledge, no *insight* into the matter; he believes he can only give himself over to the *belief* that, beyond his powers of thought, some basis or other for its validity exists.

The anthroposophical world view is in no danger of having to regard the limitations of the evidence-based method of proof as at the same time the limits of scientific conviction. It has led us to the view that the core of the world flows into our thinking, that we do not think *about* the essential being of the world, but rather that thinking is a merging with the essential being of reality. With intuition a truth is not imposed upon us from outside, because from our standpoint there *is* no inner and outer in the sense assumed by the scientific school of thought just characterized, that is in opposition to our own. For us, intuition is a direct inhabiting of things, a penetrating into the truth that gives us everything that pertains to it at all. It merges completely with what is given to us in our intuitive judgement. The essential characteristic of *faith* is totally absent here, which is that only the finished truth is given us and not its basis, and that penetrating insight into the matter under consideration is denied us. Insight gained on the path of intuition is just as scientific as insight based on external proof.

Every single organism represents the development of the *typus* into a particular form. Every organism is an individuality that governs and determines itself from a centre. It is a self-enclosed whole, which in inorganic nature is only the case with the *cosmos*.

The ideal of inorganic science is to grasp the totality of all phenomena as a unified system, so that we approach every phenomenon with the consciousness of recognizing it as a part of the cosmos. In organic science, on the other hand, in the *typus* and in its specific forms of manifestation, the ideal must be to have the greatest possible perfection in what we see *develop* through the sequence of single beings. Leading the *typus* through all the phenomena is what matters here. In inorganic science it is the *system*; in organic science it is comparison (of each individual form with the *typus*).

Spectral analysis and the perfecting of astronomy are extending out to the universe the truths gained in the more limited region of the earth. They are thereby approaching the first ideal. The second ideal will be fulfilled when *the comparative method employed by Goethe* is recognized in all its implications.

*

[...] Goethe everywhere takes the route of experience in the strictest sense. He first of all takes the objects as they are and seeks, while keeping all subjective opinions completely at a distance, to penetrate their nature; he then sets up the conditions under which the objects can enter into mutual interaction and waits to see what will result. Goethe seeks to give nature the opportunity, in particularly characteristic situations that he establishes, to bring its lawfulness into play, to express its own laws itself, as it were.

[...] For a long time people saw the only task of science as distinguishing precisely between things. We need only recall the state of affairs in which Goethe found natural history. Through Linnaeus it had become the ideal to seek precise differences between individual plants in order in this way to be able to use the most insignificant characteristics to set up new species and subspecies. Two kinds of animals or plants that differed in only the most inessential ways were assigned right away to different species. If an unexpected deviation from the arbitrarily established character of the species was found in one or another creature that until then had been assigned to a particular species, people did not then reflect how such a deviation could be explained through this character itself, but simply recorded a new species.

Making distinctions like this is the task of the intellect, which separates concepts and maintains them in this separation. This is a necessary preliminary stage of any higher scientific work. Above all, in fact, we need firmly established, clearly delineated concepts before we can seek their harmony and synthesis. But we must not remain stuck in this separation. For the intellect things are separated that humanity has an essential need to see in a harmonious unity, such as cause and effect, mechanism and organism, freedom and necessity, idea and reality, spirit and nature, and so on. All these distinctions are introduced by the intellect. They must be introduced, because otherwise the world would appear to us as a blurred, obscure chaos that would form a unity only because it would be totally undefined for us. The intellect itself is in no position to go beyond this separation.

To go beyond this is the task of reason. This has to allow the concepts created by the intellect to pass over into one another. It has to show that what the intellect keeps strictly separated is actually an inner unity. The separation is something brought about artificially, a necessary intermediary stage for our activity of knowing, not its conclusion. A person who grasps reality in a merely intellectual way distances himself from it ...

The conflict that has arisen between an intellectually

motivated science and the human heart stems from this.
Many people whose thinking is not yet developed enough
for them to arrive at a unified world view grasped in full
conceptual clarity are, nevertheless, very well able to
penetrate into the inner harmony of the universe with
their feeling. Their hearts give them what reason offers
more scientifically developed people [...]

There are sometimes difficulties in connecting the
thoughts that the intellect has created. The history of science provides us with many proofs of this. We often see
the human spirit struggle to bridge the differences created
by the intellect. [...] *Reason brings into view the higher unity
of the intellect's concepts, a unity that the intellect certainly has
in its configurations but is unable to see.* The fact that this is
overlooked is the basis of many misunderstandings about
the application of reason in the sciences.

To a small degree every science, even at its starting-
point, yes, even our everyday thinking—needs reason. If
in the judgement that every body has a specific weight we
join the subject-concept with the predicate-concept, there
already lies in this a uniting of two concepts and therefore
the simplest activity of reason.

The unity that reason takes as its object is certain *before*
all thinking,[2] before any use of reason; but it is hidden,
present only as potential, does not manifest as a fact in its
own right. Then the human spirit brings about separation,
in order, by reuniting the separate parts through reason, to
see fully into reality.

3. The Mission of Reverence

In this chapter, taken from lectures given many years later than the previous section, Steiner takes the theme of intuition and feeling as a form of true cognition one step further, and from a quite different angle. He places emphasis now on a reverent attitude to life – an attitude, of course, that many doctors would see as intrinsic to their profession.

Steiner stresses that unknown supersensible realms can be grasped by feeling before thinking comes in. It is necessary to love the unknown.

In a second passage, from a course relating to children with special needs, he speaks of love and devotion, not as vague feelings but as objective tools in the intuitive process.

While readers may question what these deliberations have to do with medicine, Steiner would see them as an essential pre-requisite, the fundamental attitude of soul without which neither medical research nor the doctor-patient relationship can benefit. Medicines must be developed through knowledge of the relationship between microcosm (the human being) and macrocosm (the world and cosmos), and this knowledge can only arise from developing faculties such as he describes. Likewise, a doctor can only diagnose and prescribe in a beneficial way based on these same faculties of intuition, reverence and love, all of which give rise to true knowledge. Steiner also here emphasizes the need for 'attention to detail' as opposed to the broad sweep of abstraction: again, a faculty that every doctor needs to develop. He speaks too of the courage and honesty required to find the right way of meeting another human being, whether handicapped child, patient or colleague.

Every good clinician will use intuition to a certain extent. However this is usually confined to the psychological level. In anthroposophical medicine it is used in the diagnosis and treatment of illness at four levels: ego, astral, etheric and physical.[1] When working with patients and remedies it is helpful to ask: 'What do I actually experience here, what strikes me about the patient?' From this insights can arise, though often not immediately. When, after careful attention to detail and meditative reflection, an insight or answer arises about the best approach with a patient, this can feel like grace – an answer from beyond oneself.

We learn about the external world through perceptions; they stimulate us to gain knowledge of our surroundings. To this end, we need only devote our attention to the outer world and not stand blankly in front of it, for then the outer world itself draws us on to satisfy our thirst for knowledge by observing it. With regard to gaining knowledge of the supersensible world, we are in a quite different situation. First of all the supersensible world is not there in front of us. If someone wishes to gain knowledge of it, so that this knowledge permeates his consciousness soul,[2] the impulse to do so must come from within and must penetrate his thinking through and through. This impulse can come only from the other powers of his soul, feeling and willing. Unless his thinking is stimulated by both these powers, it will never be impelled to approach the supersensible world. This does not mean that the supersensible is merely a feeling, but that feeling and willing must act as inner guides towards its unknown realm. What qualities, then, must feeling and willing acquire in order to do this?

First of all, someone might object to the use of a feeling as a guide to knowledge. But a simple consideration will show that in fact this is what feeling does. Anyone who takes knowledge seriously will admit that in acquiring knowledge we must proceed logically. We use logic as an instrument for testing the knowledge we acquire. How, then, if logic is this instrument, can logic itself be proved? One might say that logic can prove itself. Yes, but before we begin proving logic by logic, it must at least be possible to grasp logic with our feeling. Logical thought cannot be proved primarily by logical thought, but only by feeling. Indeed, everything that constitutes logic is first proved through feeling, by the infallible feeling for truth that dwells in the human soul. From this we can see how feeling is the foundation of logic and of thinking. Feeling must give us an impulse for the verification of thought. What must feeling become if it is to provide an impulse not only for thinking in general, but for thinking about worlds with which we are at first unacquainted and cannot survey?

Feeling of this kind must be a force which strives from within towards an object yet unknown. When the human soul seeks to encompass with feeling some other thing, we call this feeling love. Love can of course be felt for something known, and there are many things in the world for us to love. But as love is a feeling, and a feeling is the foundation of thinking in the widest sense, we must be clear that the unknown supersensible can be grasped by feeling before thinking enters in. Unprejudiced observation, accordingly, shows that it must be possible for human beings to come to love the unknown supersensible before they are able to conceive it in terms of thought. This love is indeed indispensable before the light of thought can penetrate the supersensible.

At this stage, also, the will can be permeated by a force which goes out towards the supersensible unknown. This quality of the will, which enables us to wish to carry out our aims and intentions with regard to the unknown, is devotion. The will can thus inspire devotion towards the unknown, while feeling becomes love of the unknown; and when these two emotions are united they together give rise to reverence in the true sense of the word. Then this devotion becomes the impulse that will lead us into the unknown, so that the unknown can be grasped by our thinking. Thus it is that reverence becomes the educator of the consciousness soul. For in ordinary life, also, we can say that when a person endeavours to grasp with his thinking some external reality not yet known to him, he approaches it with love and devotion. Never will the consciousness soul gain a knowledge of external objects unless love and devotion inspire its quest; otherwise the objects will not be truly observed. This also applies quite specially to all endeavours to gain knowledge of the supersensible world.

In all cases, however, the soul must allow itself to be educated by the 'I', the source of self-consciousness. We have seen how the 'I' or ego[3] gains increasing independence and strength by overcoming certain soul qualities, such as anger, and by cultivating others, such as the sense of truth. After that, the self-education of the ego comes to an end and its education through reverence begins. Anger is to be overcome and discarded; a sense of truth is to permeate the ego; reverence is to flow from the ego towards the object of which knowledge is sought. Thus, having raised itself out of the sentient soul and the intellectual soul,[4] by overcoming anger and other passions, and by cultivating a sense of truth, the ego is drawn gradually into the consciousness soul by the influence of reverence. If this reverence becomes stronger and stronger, one can speak of it as a powerful impulse towards the realm described by Goethe:

All things transient
Are but a parable;
Earth's insufficiency
Here finds fulfilment;
The indescribable
Here becomes deed;
The eternal feminine
Draws us on high.

The soul is drawn by the strength of its reverence towards the eternal, with which it longs to unite itself. But the ego has two aspects. It is impelled by necessity to continually enhance its own strength and activity. At the same time it has the task of not allowing itself to fall under the hardening influence of egotism. If the ego seeks to go further and gain knowledge of the unknown and the supersensible, and takes reverence as its guide, it is exposed to the immediate danger of losing itself. This is most likely to happen, above all, to a human being if his will is always submissive to the world. If this attitude increasingly gains the upper hand, the result may be that the ego goes out of itself and loses itself in the other being or thing to which it has submitted. This condition can be likened to fainting by the soul, as distinct from bodily fainting. In bodily fainting the ego sinks into undefined darkness. In fainting of the soul, the ego loses itself spiritually while the bodily faculties and perceptions of the outer world are not impaired. This can happen if the ego is not strong enough to extend itself fully into the will and to guide it.

This self-surrender by the ego can be the final result of a systematic mortification of the will. A person who pursues this course becomes incapable of willing or acting on his own account; he has surrendered his will to the object of his submissive devotion and has lost his own self. When this condition prevails, it produces an enduring impotence of the soul. Only when a devotional feeling is warmed through by the ego, so that a person can immerse himself in it without losing his ego, can it be salutary for the human soul.

How, then, can reverence always carry the ego with it? The ego cannot allow itself to be led in any direction, as human self, unless it maintains in its thinking a knowledge of itself. Nothing else can protect the ego from losing itself when devotion leads it out into the world. The soul can be led out of itself towards something external by the force of will, but when the soul leaves behind the boundary of the external, it must make sure of being illuminated by the light of thought.

Thinking itself cannot lead the soul out; this comes about through devotion. But thinking must then immediately exert itself to permeate with thought the object of the soul's devotion. In other words, there must be a resolve to think about this object. Directly the devotional impulse loses the will to think, there is a danger of losing oneself. If anyone makes it a matter of principle not to think about the object of his devotion, this can lead in extreme cases to a lasting debility of the soul.

Is love, the other element in reverence, subject to a similar fate? Something that radiates from the human self towards the unknown must be poured into love, so that never for a moment does the ego fail to sustain itself. The ego must have the will to enter into everything which forms the object of its devotion, and it must maintain itself in face of the external, the unknown, the supersensible. What becomes of love if the ego fails to maintain itself at the moment of encountering the unknown, if it is unwilling to bring the light of thinking and of rational judgement to bear on the unknown? Love of that kind becomes mere sentimental enthusiasm. But the ego can begin to find its way from the intellectual soul, where it lives, to the external unknown, and then it can never extinguish itself altogether. Unlike the will, the ego cannot completely mortify itself. When the soul seeks to embrace the external world with feeling, the ego is always present in the feeling, but if it is not supported by thinking and willing, it rushes forth without restraint, unconscious of itself. And if this love for the unknown is not accompanied by resolute thinking, the soul can fall into a sentimental extreme, somewhat like sleep-walking, just as the state reached by the soul when submissive devotion leads to loss of the self is somewhat like a bodily fainting-fit. When a sentimental enthusiast goes forth to encounter the unknown, he leaves behind the strength of the ego and takes with him only secondary forces. Since the strength of the ego is absent from his consciousness, he tries to grasp the unknown as one does in the realm of dreams. Under these conditions the soul falls into what may be called an enduring state of dreaming or somnambulism.

Again, if the soul is unable to relate itself properly to the world and to other people, if it rushes out into life and shrinks from using the light of thought to illuminate its situation, then the ego, having fallen into a somnambulistic condition, is bound to go astray and to wander through the world like a will-o'-the-wisp.

If the soul succumbs to mental laziness and shuns the

light of thought when it meets the unknown, then, and only then, will it harbour superstitions in one or other form. The sentimental soul, with its fond dreams, wandering through life as though asleep, and the indolent soul, unwilling to be fully conscious of itself — these are the souls most inclined to believe everything blindly. Their tendency is to avoid the effort of thinking for themselves and to allow truth and knowledge to be prescribed for them.

If we are to get to know an external object, we have to bring our own productive thinking to bear on it, and it is the same with the supersensible, whatever form this may take. Never, in seeking to gain a knowledge of the supersensible, must we exclude thinking. Directly we rely on merely observing the supersensible, we are exposed to all possible deceptions and errors. All such errors and superstitions, all the wrong or untruthful ways of entering the supersensible worlds, can be attributed in the last instance to a refusal to allow consciousness to be illuminated by the light of creative thought. No one can be deceived by information said to come from the spiritual world if he has the will to keep his thinking always active and independent. Nothing else will suffice, and this is something that every spiritual researcher will confirm. The stronger the will is in creative thinking, the greater is the possibility of gaining true, clear and certain knowledge of the spiritual world.

Thus we see the need for a means of education which will lead the ego into the consciousness soul and will guide the consciousness soul in the face of the unknown, both the physical unknown and the unknown super-sensible. Reverence, consisting of devotion and love, provides the means we seek. When the latter are imbued with the right kind of self-aware feeling, they become steps which lead to ever greater heights.

True devotion, in whatever form it is experienced by the soul, whether through prayer or otherwise, can never lead us astray. The best way of learning to know something is to approach it first of all with love and devotion. A healthy education will consider especially how strength can be given to the development of the soul through the de-votional impulse. To a child the world is largely unknown. If we are to guide him towards knowledge and sound judgement of it, the best way is to awaken in him a feeling of reverence towards it; and we can be sure that by so doing we shall lead him to fullness of experience in any walk of life.

It is very important for the human soul if it can look back to a childhood in which devotion, leading on to reverence, was often felt. Frequent opportunities to look up to revered persons, and to gaze with heartfelt devotion at things that are still beyond its understanding, provide a good impulse for higher development in later life. A person will always gratefully remember those occasions when, as a child in the family circle, he heard of some outstanding personality of whom everyone spoke with devotion and reverence. A feeling of holy awe, which gives reverence a specially intimate character, will then permeate the soul. Or someone may relate how with trembling hand, later on, he rang the bell and shyly made his way into the room of the revered personality whom he was meeting for the first time, after having heard him spoken of with so much respectful admiration. Simply to have come into his presence and exchanged a few words can confirm a devotion which will be particularly helpful when we are trying to unravel the great riddles of existence and are seeking for the goal which we long to make our own. Here reverence is a force that draws us upwards, and by so doing fortifies and invigorates the soul.

How can this be? Let us consider the outward expression of reverence in human gestures — what forms does it take? We bend our knees, fold our hands, and incline our heads towards the object of our reverence. These are the organs whereby the ego, and above all the higher faculties of the soul, can express themselves most intensively.

*

How can you learn to perceive such facts for yourselves? You can find your way to such perceptions if you set out to do so with the love that I have described to you and upon which you will remember I laid such stress. You must never say: 'In order to perceive such things, I should have to be clairvoyant.' To say that betokens an inner laziness — a quality that must on no account ever be found in one who undertakes the task of education. Long before you attain to the clairvoyance that is required for spiritual research in general, for instance, you can develop in yourself the faculty simply to perceive what is really in front of you. The power to do this can be born in you if you approach with loving devotion all that shows itself in the child, and especially those very developments that accompany abnormal conditions. What you say to yourself at such a moment will be true. There is of course need here for esoteric courage. This esoteric courage can and does develop in man—provided only that one thing does not stand in the way.

It is strange, and at the same time significant, that these inner intuitions are so little noticed by people who are, comparatively speaking, well able to have them. Anthroposophists have many opportunities to pay heed to such inner intuitions! For they *have* these intuitions, far more than is supposed, but they fail to attend to them—the reason being that, in the moment when they should do so, they find themselves assailed by a *vanity* that is hard to overcome. With the discovery of faculties not known before, all manner of impulses that spring from vanity begin to crop up in the soul. Along with the other characteristics of our age that I described for you in my lecture yesterday, as well as on several other occasions, we have also to reckon with a tendency to grow vain and conceited, for it is a tendency that is terribly prevalent in modern mankind.

This is a matter that should receive serious consideration from those of the youth of today—you yourselves of course included—who are devoting their lives to some great and noble calling. There is in our time great need for young men and women to rise up among us and exercise a regenerating influence upon mankind. And what I am now going to say is not said out of misunderstanding of the youth movement of our day, nor from lack of understanding, but out of a true understanding of it. It is a necessity, this youth movement, it is something of quite extraordinary significance; and for those older people who can understand it, the modern youth movement is interesting in the highest degree. Not a word shall be uttered here against it. Nor shall we attempt to deny that there is only too often a deplorable lack of readiness on the part of the older generation to understand this youth movement, and that a great many plans have been wrecked just because the movement has not been taken seriously enough, just because people have not troubled themselves to look into it sufficiently. But the youth movement does need to beware of one thing when it sets out to undertake specific practical tasks; and it is incumbent on those of us who have had experience in the matter to call attention to it, for it presents a great problem for the whole future of the movement. I mean a certain vanity that is very prevalent.

This vanity is not so much due to a lack of manners, but is rather the consequence of a situation that may well be inevitable. For the will to action necessitates of course a strong development of inner capacities, and then it follows all too easily that under the influence of Ahriman vanity begins to spring up in the soul. I have had opportunity in my life to make careful and intimate observation

of persons who were full of promise—persons too of the
most various ages—in whom one could see again and
again how with the dawn of the age that has followed Kali
Yuga[5] vanity began to grow and thrive in their souls. It is
not, therefore, only among young people that vanity
shows itself. What concerns us at the moment, however, is
the special form of it that manifests in them, and that has
in point of fact hindered them from developing the right
and essential character that lies inherent in being young
today, waiting to be developed. Hence the phenomenon
with which we are so familiar, this endless talk of 'mis-
sions', of great tasks, with all too little inclination to set to
work upon the details, to take pains about the *small* things
that require to be done in carrying out these tasks.

In the future there will be great need for what has been
described in an extraordinarily middle-class context, but
also with a degree of intuition, as *devotion to detail.* Devotion to detail and to little things is something which the
youth of our time need to develop. They are far too apt to
revel in abstractions; and this revelling in abstractions is
the very thing that can then lure them with irresistible
force into the snare of vanity. I do beg you to consider the
difficulties that beset your path on this account. Make it a
matter of esoteric striving to master this tendency to
vanity; for it does indeed constitute a real hindrance to
any work you undertake.

Suppose you want to be able to speak to some fellow
human being out of an intuitive power of vision. The
things you need to behold in him are by no means written

plain for all to see, and you may take it that statements made about handicapped children from the ordinary lay point of view are generally false. What you have to do is to see *through* what lies on the surface, see right through it to the real state of affairs. If therefore you want to come to the point of being able to say something to him out of intuitive perception, what do you need for that? You need to tell yourself with courage and with energy, not just saying it at some particular moment but carrying it continually in your consciousness so that it determines the very quality and content of your consciousness: 'I can do it.' If, without vanity, in a spirit of self-sacrifice and in earnest endeavour to overcome all the things that hinder, you repeat these words, not only feeling them, but saying them to yourself over and over again, then you will begin to discover how far you are able to go in this direction. Do not expect to find the development of the faculty you seek by spinning out all manner of theories and thoughts. No, what you need to do is to maintain all the time this courageous consciousness, which develops quite simply of itself when once you have begun to fetch up from the depths of your soul what lies hidden there, buried (metaphorically speaking) beneath dirt and swamp and peat bog.

But, my dear friends, meditation that employs such pictures as I have been giving can never take its course in the kind of mood that would allow us to feel: 'Now I am going to settle down to a blissful time of meditation; it will be like sinking into a snug, warm nest!' No, the feeling must be continually present in us that we are taking the plunge into *reality*—that we are grasping hold of reality.

Devotion to little things—yes, to the very smallest of all! We must not omit to cultivate this interest in very little things. The ear lobe, the paring of a finger-nail, a single human hair—should be every bit as interesting to us as Saturn, sun and moon. For really and truly in one human hair everything else is comprised; a person who becomes bald loses a whole cosmos! What we see externally we can verily create inwardly, if only we achieve that overcoming of ourselves which is essential to a life of meditation. But we shall never achieve it so long as any vestige of vanity is allowed to remain—and vestiges of vanity lurk in every corner and crevice of the soul. Therefore it is so urgent, my dear friends, if you want to become real educators, and especially educators of handicapped children, that you should cultivate, with the utmost humility, this devotion to small things. And when you have made a beginning in this way in your own sphere, you can afterwards go on to awaken in other circles of the youth movement this same devotion to little things.

And then it will indeed become possible for you to receive, for example, indications that are afterwards verified from external evidence—as happened, you remember, in the case we are considering. And here I must say in connection with this very case, I have often occasion to find grave fault in connection with the various under-takings that have started within our anthroposophical movement. The situation was as follows. Here was a girl concerning whom I told you that a kind of abnormality must have occurred in her development between the third and fourth year. You questioned the mother, and the mother confirmed that it was so. What did you do then? Please tell me, honestly and sincerely: what did you do, when the mother confirmed the fact? [Silence.] Please be esoterically honest and tell me the truth, you three: what did you do? [Silence.] If you had done the right thing, you would now be telling me: 'We danced and jumped until we made a hole in the ceiling!' And the after-effect of this jumping for joy would still be expressing itself today — and not merely in words, it would be shining out from you like a light.

That is what you need — *enthusiasm in the experience of truth*. This enthusiasm is an absolute *sine qua non*. For years it has been so terribly painful to me, the way the members of the anthroposophical movement stand there as if they were rooted to the spot — and the young too, almost as much as the old. But now consider what it *means*, that they can stand there so impassively. Look at Nietzsche! What a different sort of fellow he was — even if he did get ill from it! He made his Zarathustra become a dancer. Can't you become dancers — in the sense Nietzsche meant it? Why, you should be leading lives of joy — deep inner joy in the truth! There is nothing in the world more delightful, nothing more fascinating, than the experience of truth. There you have an esotericism that is far more genuine, far more significant than the esotericism that goes about with a long face. Before everything else—and long before you begin to talk about having a 'mission'—there must be this living inner experience of truth.

4. The Four Temperaments

The following passages examine the supersensible bodies (etheric, astral and ego) from various viewpoints. Steiner describes the four temperaments — choleric, sanguine, phlegmatic and melancholic — as mediating between our eternal individuality and physical heredity. Since they have a link with physical attributes as well as soul qualities, they are very accessible to experience and therefore a good starting-point for approaching aspects of the human being that cannot be quantified in the same way as bodily processes. While these four categories may initially appear schematic, Steiner points out that they invariably combine and intermingle in each of us, with one temperament predominating. They are therefore tendencies rather than fixed types, and a useful, flexible diagnostic tool in understanding ourselves and others.

The choleric

Steiner says that in this temperament the ego predominates, expressed physically through the blood. Let us try to reproduce in ourselves a choleric mood. What observations can we make? It certainly has to do with wanting to get things done, possibly in a somewhat aggressive manner. We also get more in touch with our identity, with a true kernel of our being. When a more phlegmatic person becomes choleric, he is said to 'show a bit of spirit' that otherwise remains dormant. The spirit is a manifestation of the ego. During a choleric outburst most people get flushed, the pulse rate increases and the blood pressure rises, and they might suffer from palpitations. Cholerics are hot-blooded people. Thus one can understand that the choleric temperament connects us to our identity on the one hand and works in our blood and circulation on the other.

The sanguine

Steiner says that the astral body (soul) predominates in this temperament, and is physically expressed in the nervous system. It is not immediately obvious why this is so. Let us be sanguine for a while. We enjoy talking and often talk about anything that comes into our head, constantly changing the subject as one idea associates with another. When relating an experience we are filled with the intense emotion that the experience originally called forth. Sanguine people are invariably wide-awake and very open to sense impressions such as sound and smell. When under stress they can become a bag of nerves, jumping at the tiniest noise. We can thus understand the strong connections this temperament has with the nervous system. The astral is the body of feeling and movement (a key characteristic of the animal kingdom). As shown in the text, the ego is needed to guard against the astral body's excesses. I once had a patient who developed acute psychosis when she became anaemic (i.e., her blood and ego forces were weakened). This resolved as soon as her haemoglobin returned to normal, thus illustrating what Steiner refers to here.

The phlegmatic

According to Steiner, the etheric body predominates in the phlegmatic temperament and is expressed physically in the glandular system. Let us slip in to the phlegmatic temperament for a moment. We continually want to indulge in our creature comforts, such as a good meal and the feeling of well-being that a post-prandial stupour produces. This is when all the digestive glands are fully at work. Phlegmatics are not averse to enjoying vegetative periods, revealing their kinship to the plant kingdom. As phlegmatics we are not so keen on excitement as the sanguine, neither are we desperate for action like the choleric; instead we are quite happy to stay put in one place – again demonstrating a connection to the plant world. We develop a different relation-ship to time, finding that most things can actually wait a while.

Steiner tells us that when we fall sleep the ego and astral move into the spirit world, while the physical and etheric are left in bed. Growth mainly takes place at night, when the etheric is free from the inhibiting influence of the higher bodies. Growth is of course another basic feature of plants and is influenced by glandular secretions, e.g. growth hormones. The reproductive system, which has a strong connection to the etheric, is also very much under the influence of glandular secretions.

The melancholic

Steiner says that the physical body predominates in the melancholic temperament. To understand the melancholic we need to feel the weight of the physical body. Everything is an effort. Small bodily complaints often loom large. Melancholics are more prone to degenerative illnesses, suggesting a connection to the physical. They can also have great understanding for the suffering of others, however.

We can distinguish a confluence of two streams, of which each human being is composed: on the one hand what comes to us from our family, and on the other hand what has developed from our innermost being, i.e., a number of predispositions, characteristics, inner capacities and outer destiny.[1] These must be reconciled. We find that a person must adapt himself to this union in accordance with his innermost being on the one hand, and on the other in accordance with what is brought to him from the line of heredity. We see how a person bears to a great degree the physiognomy of his ancestors. We could put him together, as it were, from the sum of his various ancestors. Since at first the inner essential kernel has nothing to do with what is inherited, but must merely adapt itself to what is most suitable to it, we shall see that it is necessary for a certain mediation to exist for what has lived perhaps for centuries in an entirely different world and is now again transplanted into another world. The spirit being of man must have something here below to which it is related. There must be a bond, a connecting link, between the special individual human being and humanity in general, into which he is born through family, people, race.

Between these two, namely, what we bring with us from our earlier life and what our family, ancestors and race imprint upon us, there is a mediation, something that bears more general characteristics but at the same time is capable of being individualized. What occupies this position between the line of heredity and the line which represents our individuality is expressed by the word temperament. In what confronts us in the temperament of a person we have something in a certain way like a physiognomy of his innermost individuality. We thus understand how the individuality colours by means of the qualities of temperament the attributes inherited in the succession of generations. Temperament stands in the middle between what we bring with us as individuals and what originates from the line of heredity. When the two streams unite, the one stream colours the other. They colour each other reciprocally. Just as blue and yellow, let us say, unite in green, so do the two streams in man unite in what we call temperament. Our temperament is everything that mediates between all inner characteristics that we bring with us from our earlier incarnation on the one hand and, on the other, what the line of heredity endows us with. It takes its place between the inherited characteristics and what we have absorbed into our inner essential being. It is as if upon its descent to earth this kernel of being were to envelop itself with a spiritual nuance of what awaits it here below, so that in proportion as this kernel of being is able best to adapt itself to this physical covering for the human being, the kernel of being colours itself according to what it is born into and to a quality that it brings with it. Here shine forth the soul qualities of man and his natural inherited attributes. Between the two is the temperament — between what connects a person with his ancestors and what he brings with him from his earlier incarnations. The temperament balances the eternal with the transitory.

This balancing occurs through the fact that what we call the 'members' or bodily sheaths[2] of human nature come into relation with one another in a quite definite way. We understand this in detail, however, only when we place before our mind's eye the complete human being as spiritual science sees him. Only through spiritual science can the mystery of the human temperament be discovered.

We find that this human being formed by the merging of these two streams is a fourfold being. So we shall be able to say when we consider the entire individual that the human being consists of *the physical body, the etheric body* or *body of formative forces*, *the astral body* and *the ego*.

In that part of man perceptible to the outer senses, which is all that materialistic thought is willing to recognize, we have first, according to spiritual science, only one part of the human being, the physical body, which man has in common with the mineral world. The part subject to physical laws is something we have in common with all nature, the sum of chemical and physical laws.

Beyond this, however, we recognize higher super-sensible members of human nature that are as actual and essential as the outer physical body. As first supersensible member, man has the etheric body, which becomes part of his organism and remains united with the physical body throughout his entire life; only at death does a separation of the two take place. Even this first supersensible member of human nature, in spiritual science called the etheric or life body (we might also call it the glandular body), is no more visible to our outer eyes than are colours to those born blind. But it exists, actually and perceptibly exists, for what Goethe calls the eyes of the spirit, and it is even more real than the outer physical body because it is the builder, the moulder, of the physical body. During the entire time between birth and death this etheric or life body con-tinuously combats the disintegration of the physical body. Any kind of mineral product of nature—a crystal, for example—is so constituted that it is permanently held together by its own forces, by the forces of its own sub-stance. That is not the case with the physical body of a living being. Here the physical forces work in such a way that they destroy the form of life, as we are able to observe after death when physical forces destroy the life-form. That this destruction does not occur during life, that the physical body does not conform to the physical and chemical forces and laws, is due to the fact that the etheric or life body is ceaselessly combating these forces.

The third member of the human being we recognize in the bearer of all pleasure and suffering, joy and pain, instincts, impulses, passions, desires and all that surges to and fro as sensations and ideas, even all concepts of what we designate as moral ideals, and so on. That we call the astral body. Do not take exception to this expression. We could also call it the 'nerve-body'. Spiritual science sees in it something real and knows indeed that this body of impulses and desires is not an effect of the physical body but the cause of this body. It knows that the soul-spiritual part has built up for itself the physical body.

Thus we already have three members of the human being. As man's highest member we recognize something that enables him to tower above all other beings, by means of which he is the crown of earth's creation, namely, the bearer of the human ego, which gives him in such a mysterious but also in such a manifest way the powers of self-consciousness.

Man has the physical body in common with his entire visible environment, the etheric body in common with the plants and animals, the astral body with the animals. The fourth member, however, the ego, he has for himself alone, and by means of it he towers above the other visible creatures on earth. We recognize this fourth member as the ego-bearer, as that in human nature by means of which man is able to say 'I' to himself, to come to independence.

Now what we see physically, and what the intellect that is bound to the physical senses can know, is only an expression of these four members of the human being. Thus, the expression of the ego, of the actual ego-bearer, is the blood in it circulation. This very special fluid is the expression of the ego. The physical sense expression of the astral body in man is, for example, among other things, the nervous system. The expression of the etheric body, or a part of this expression, is the glandular system. The physical body expresses itself in the sense organs. These four members confront us in the human being. So when we observe the complete human being we shall be able to say that he consists of physical body, etheric body, astral body and ego. What is primarily physical body, which the human being bears in such a way that it is visible to physical eyes, clearly bears, first of all, when viewed from without, the marks of heredity. Also those characteristics that live in man's etheric body (which combats disintegration of the physical body) come from the line of heredity. Then we come to his astral body, whose characteristics are much more closely bound to the essential kernel of the human being. If we turn to this innermost kernel, to the actual ego, we find what passes from incarnation to incarnation and appears as an inner mediator that rays forth its essential qualities. Now in the whole human being all the separate members work into each other; they act reciprocally. Because two streams flow together in man when he enters the physical world, there arises a fluctuating combination of man's four members, in which one gains mastery over the others, impressing its colour upon them. Now according to which of these members comes especially into prominence, the individual develops this or that temperament. The particular colouring of human nature, what we call the actual shade of the temperament, depends upon whether the forces, the different means of power, of one member or of another predominate, have a preponderance over the others. Man's eternal being, which goes from incarnation to incarnation,[3] so expresses itself in each new embodiment that it calls forth a certain reciprocal action among the four members of human nature—the ego, astral body, etheric body and physical body—and from the interaction of these four members arises the colouring of human nature that we characterize as temperament.

When the essential being has tinged the physical and etheric bodies, what arises because of the colouring thus given will act upon each of the other members. So that the way an individual appears to us with his characteristics depends upon whether the inner kernel acts more strongly upon the physical body or whether, on the contrary, the physical body acts more strongly upon our inner core. The human being is able according to his nature to influence one of the four members [physical, etheric, astral, ego], and through the reaction of this upon the other members our temperament originates. When our essential core of individuality comes into re-embodiment, it is able to introduce into one or another of its members a certain surplus of activity. Thus it can give to the ego a certain surplus strength. Or again, the individual can influence his other members as a result of having had certain experiences in his former life.

When the ego of an individual has become so strong through its destiny that its forces are noticeably dominant in fourfold human nature and it dominates the other members, then the *choleric* temperament results. If a person is especially subject to the influence of the forces of the astral body, then he develops a *sanguine* temperament. If the etheric or life body acts excessively upon a person, the *phlegmatic* temperament comes about. And when the physical body with its laws is especially predominant in the human nature, so that the spiritual essence of being is not able to overcome a certain hardness in the physical body, then we have to do with the *melancholic* temperament. Just as the eternal and the transitory intermingle, so does the relation of the members to one another arise in dynamic interaction.

I have already told you how the four members of our being [*physical, etheric, astral, ego*] express themselves outwardly in the physical body. Thus, a large part of the physical body is the direct expression of the human physical life principle. The physical body as such comes to expression only in the physical body. Thus it is the physical body that gives the keynote in a *melancholic*.

We must regard the glandular system as the physical expression of the etheric body. The etheric body expresses itself physically in the glandular system. Hence in a *phlegmatic* person the glandular system gives the keynote to the physical body.

The nervous system and, of course, what occurs through it we must regard as the physical expression of the astral body. The astral body finds its physical expression in the nervous system. Therefore in a *sanguine* person the nervous system gives the keynote to the physical body.

The blood in its circulation, the force of the pulsation of the blood, is the expression of the actual ego. The ego expresses itself in the circulation of the blood, in the predominating activity of the blood. It shows itself especially in the fiery, vehement blood. One must try to penetrate more subtly into the connection that exists between the ego and the other members of the human being. Suppose, for example, the ego exerts a particular force in the life of sensations, ideas and the nervous system. Suppose that in the case of a certain person everything arises from his ego, everything that he feels he feels strongly, because his ego is strong. We call that the choleric temperament. What has received its character from the ego will make itself felt as the predominating quality. Hence in a *choleric* the blood system is predominant.

The choleric temperament will show itself as active in strongly pulsating blood. In this the element of force in the individual makes its appearance in the fact that he has a special influence upon his blood. In such a person, in whom spiritually the ego and physically the blood is particularly active, we see the innermost force vigorously keeping the organization fit. And as he thus confronts the outer world, the force of his ego will wish to make itself felt. That is the effect of this ego. By reason of this, the choleric appears as one who wishes to assert his ego in all circumstances. All the aggressiveness of the choleric, everything connected with his strong will-nature, may be ascribed to the circulation of the blood.

When the astral body predominates in an individual, the physical expression of this will lie in the functions of the nervous system, that instrument of the rising and falling waves of sensation. And what the astral body accomplishes is the life of thoughts, of images, so that the person who is endowed with the sanguine temperament will have the predisposition to live in the surging sensations and feelings and in the images of his life of ideas. We must understand clearly the relation of the astral body to the ego. The astral body functions between the nervous system and the blood system. So it is perfectly clear what this relation is. If the sanguine temperament were the only one present, if only the nervous system were active, being quite especially prominent as the expression of the astral body, then such a person would have a life of shifting images and ideas. In this way a chaos of images would come and go. He would be given over to all the restless flux of sensations, from image to image, from idea to idea. Something of that sort appears if the astral body predominates, that is, in a sanguine person who in a certain sense is given over to the tide of sensations, images, etc., since in him the astral body and the nervous system predominate. It is the forces of the ego that prevent the images from darting about in a fantastic way. Only because these images are controlled by the ego does harmony and order enter in. Were man not to check them with his ego, they would surge up and down without any evidence of control by the individual.

In the physical body it is the blood that principally limits the activity of the nervous system. Man's blood circulation, the blood flowing in us, is what lays fetters, as it were, upon what has its expression in the nervous system. It restrains surging feelings and sensations. It combats nerve-life. It would lead too far afield if I were to show you in all details how the nervous system and the blood are related, and how the blood is the restrainer of this life of ideas. What occurs if this restraint is not present, if a person is deficient in red blood, is anaemic? Well, even if we do not go into the most minute psychological details, from the simple fact that when a person's blood becomes too thin, that is, has a deficiency of red corpuscles, he is easily given over to the unrestrained surging back and forth of all kinds of fantastic images, even to illusion and hallucination—you can still conclude from this simple fact that the blood is the restrainer of the nervous system. A balance must exist between the ego and the astral body—or speaking physiologically, between the blood and the nervous system—so that one does not become a slave of one's nervous system, that is, of the surging life of sensation and feeling.

If now the astral body has a certain excess of activity, if there is a predominance of the astral body and its expression, the nervous system is still restrained by the blood to be sure but is not completely able to establish a condition of absolute balance, and that peculiar condition arises in which human life easily arouses an individual's interest in something, yet such interest quickly flags and passes to something else. Such a person cannot stay with an idea and in consequence his interest can be immediately kindled in everything that meets him in the outer world, but restraint is not applied to make this inwardly enduring. The interest that has been kindled quickly evaporates. In this quick kindling of interest and quick passing from one subject to another we see the expression of the predominating astral element, the sanguine temperament. The sanguine person cannot linger with an impression. He cannot hold fast to an image, cannot fix his attention upon one subject but hurries from one life impression to another, from perception to perception, from idea to idea. He shows a fickle disposition. That can be especially observed in sanguine children, and in this case it may cause one anxiety. Interest is easily aroused. A picture begins easily to have an effect, quickly makes an impression, but the impression soon vanishes again.

When there is a strong predominance in an individual of the etheric or life body, which inwardly regulates the processes of man's life and growth, and brings about a feeling of inner well-being or of discomfort, then such a person will be tempted to wish to remain in this feeling of inner comfort. The etheric body is a body that leads a sort of inner life, while the astral body expresses itself in outer interests. The ego is the bearer of our activity and will directed outwards. If this etheric body, which acts as life-sustaining body and maintains disparate functions in equilibrium, an equilibrium that expresses itself in the feeling of life's general *comfort* – when this self-sustained inner life, which chiefly causes the sense of inner comfort, predominates, then it may happen that an individual lives chiefly in this feeling of inner comfort. He may then have such a feeling of well-being when everything in his organism is in order that he feels little urgency to direct his inner being towards the outer world, is little inclined to develop a strong will. The more inwardly comfortable he feels, the more harmony will he create between the inner and outer. When this is the case, when it is even carried to excess, we have to do with a phlegmatic person.

In a melancholic we have seen that the physical body, that is, the densest member of the human being, rules the others. A person must be master of his physical body, as he must be master of a machine if he wishes to use it. But when this densest part rules, the person always feels that he is not master of it, that he cannot manage it, for the physical body is the instrument that he should rule completely through his higher members. Now, however, this physical body has dominion and sets up opposition to the others, and in this case the person concerned is not able to use his instrument perfectly, so that the other principles experience restriction because of it and disharmony exists between the physical body and the other members. This is the way the hardened physical system appears when it overbears to excess. The person is not able to bring about flexibility where it should exist. The inner human being has no power over his physical system; he feels inner obstacles. These show themselves through the fact that the person is compelled to direct his strength towards these inner obstacles. What cannot be overcome is what causes sorrow and pain, and these make it impossible for the individual to look out upon his contemporary world in an unprejudiced way. This constraint becomes a source of inner grief, which is felt as pain and sorrow. Certain thoughts and ideas begin to be enduring. The person becomes gloomy, melancholic. There is a constant sense of pain. This mood is caused by nothing else than that the physical body sets up opposition to the inner ease of the etheric body, to the mobility of the astral body, and to the ego's certainty of its goal.

If we thus comprehend the nature of the temperaments through sound knowledge, many things in life will become clear to us, but it will also become possible to handle in a practical way what we otherwise could not [...] We need only observe how the temperament comes to expression externally, in an outer picture as it were.

Let us, for instance, take the choleric person, who has a strong, firm centre in his inner being. If the ego pre-dominates, the person will assert himself against all outer oppositions. He wants to be in evidence. This ego is the restrainer. The physical body is formed according to its etheric body, the etheric body according to its astral body. This astral body would fashion man, so to speak, in the most differentiated way. But because such growth is opposed by the ego through its blood forces, balance is maintained between abundant [*etheric*] and differentiated [*astral*] growth. So when there is a surplus of ego, growth can be retarded. It positively retards the growth of the other members. It does not allow the astral body and the etheric body their full rights. In the choleric temperament you are able to recognize clearly in outer growth, in all that confronts us outwardly, the expression or picture of what is inwardly active, the actual deep inner ego-forces at work in the person. Choleric people appear as a rule as if growth had been retarded. You can find in life example after example of this, for instance the German choleric philosopher Johann Gottlieb Fichte. Even in external appearance he is recognizable as such, since in his outer form he gave the impression of being retarded in growth. Thereby he reveals clearly that the other members of his being have been held back by excess of ego. Not the astral body with its forming capacity is the predominant member, but the ego rules, the restrainer, the limiter of formative forces. Hence we see as a rule in those who are pre-eminently people of strong will, where the ego restrains the free formative force of the astral body, a small compact figure. Take another classical example of the choleric, Napoleon, the 'little General' who remained so small because the ego held back the other members of his being. There you have the type of retarded growth of the choleric. There you can see how this force of the ego works out of the spirit so that the innermost being is manifest in the outer form.

Observe the physiognomy of the choleric! Compare it with the phlegmatic person! How indefinite are his features. How little reason there is to say that such a form of forehead is suited to the choleric. One particular organ shows especially clearly whether the astral body or the ego is predominant, that is the eye, in the steady, assured aspect of the eye of the choleric. As a rule we see how this strongly kindled inner light, which turns everything luminously inwards, sometimes is expressed in a black, a coal-black eye, because, according to a certain law, the choleric does not permit the astral body to colour that very thing that his ego-force draws inwards, although it is coloured in another person. Observe such an individual in his whole bearing. An experienced observer can almost tell from the rear view whether a certain person is a choleric. The firm walk proclaims the choleric, and even in the step we see the expression of strong ego-force. In the choleric child we already notice the firm tread. When he walks on the ground, he not only sets his foot on it but he treads as if he wanted to go a little bit farther into the ground.

The overall human individual is a copy or reflection of this innermost being, which declares itself to us in such a way. Naturally, it is not a question of my maintaining that the choleric person is short and the sanguine tall. We may compare the form of a person only with his own growth. It depends upon the relation of a person's growth to the entire form.

Now turn to the sanguine person. Observe the sanguine child's glance. It quickly lights upon something but just as quickly turns to something else. It is a merry glance; an inner joy and gaiety shine in it. In it is expressed what comes from the depths of human nature, from the mobile astral body, which predominates in the sanguine person. In its mobile inner life this astral body will work upon the other members, and it will also make the person's external appearance as flexible as possible. Indeed, we are able to recognize the entire outer physiognomy, the permanent form and also the gestures, as the expression of the mobile, volatile, fluid astral body. The astral body has the tendency to fashion, to form. The inner reveals itself outwardly. Hence the sanguine person is slender and supple. Even in the slender form, the bony structure, we see the inner mobility of this astral body in the whole person. It comes to expression for example in the slim muscles. It is also to be seen in a person's external expression. Even one who is not clairvoyant can recognize from the rear whether a person is of sanguine or choleric temperament; and to be able to do this one need not be a spiritual scientist. In a sanguine person we have elastic and springing walk, in the hopping, dancing walk of the sanguine child we see the expression of the mobile astral body. The sanguine temperament manifests itself especially strongly in childhood. See how the formative tendency is expressed there, and even more delicate attributes are to be found in the outer form. Where in the choleric person we have sharply cut facial features, in the sanguine they are mobile, expressive, changeable. Likewise there appears in the sanguine child a certain inner possibility to alter his countenance. Even from the colour of the eyes we could confirm the expression of the sanguine person. The inwardness of ego-nature, the self-sufficient inwardness of the choleric meets us in his black eyes. Look at the sanguine person in whom the ego-nature is not so deep-rooted, in whom the astral body pours forth all its mobility — there the blue eye is predominant. These blue eyes are closely connected with the individual's invisible inner light, the light of the astral body.

Thus many attributes could be pointed out which reveal the temperament in external appearance. Through the four-membered human nature we learn to understand clearly this soul riddle of the temperaments. Indeed, a knowledge of the four temperaments, springing from a profound perception of human nature, has been handed down to us from ancient times. If we thus understand human nature, and know that the external is only the expression of the spiritual, then we learn to understand man in his relation even to the externalities, to understand him in his whole process of becoming. We learn to recognize what we must do concerning ourself and the child as far as temperament is concerned. In education, especially, notice must be taken of the kind of temperament that tends to develop in the child. In ordinary life and also education, an actual living knowledge of the nature of the temperaments is indispensable, and both would profit infinitely from it.

Now let us go further. We can also see how the phlegmatic temperament is brought to expression in outer form. In this temperament there predominates the activity of the etheric body, which has its physical expression in the glandular system and its soul expression in a feeling of ease, in inner balance. If in such a person everything is not only in a normal state of inner balance but, beyond this normality, these inner formative forces of ease are especially active, then their products are added to the human body. It becomes corpulent, it expands. In the largeness of the body, in development of the fatty parts, we see what the inner formative forces of the etheric body are especially working on. The inner sense of ease of the phlegmatic person meets us in all that. Who would not recognize in this lack of reciprocal action between the inner and the outer the cause of the often slovenly, dragging gait of the phlegmatic person, whose step will often not adapt itself to the ground. He does not step properly, so to speak; he does not put himself in relation to things. That he has little control over the forms of his inner being you can observe in the whole person. The phlegmatic temperament confronts one in the immobile, indifferent countenance, even in the peculiarly dull, colourless appearance of the eye. While the eye of the choleric is fiery and sparkling, we can recognize in that of the phlegmatic the expression of the etheric body, focused only upon inner ease.

The melancholic is one who cannot completely attain mastery over the physical instrument, one to whom the physical instrument offers resistance, one who cannot cope with the use of this instrument. Look at the melancholic, how he generally has a drooping head, does not have the force in himself to stiffen his neck. The bowed head shows that the inner forces that adjust the head perpendicularly are never able to unfold freely. The glance is downwards, the eye sad, unlike the black gleam of the choleric eye. We see in the peculiar appearance of the eye that the physical instrument makes difficulties for him. The walk, to he sure, is measured, firm, but not like the walk of the choleric, the firm tread of the choleric. Here it has a certain kind of dragging firmness.

All this can be only briefly indicated here, but the life of the human being will be much more understandable to us if we work in this way, if we see the spirit activating outer forms in such a way that the external part of the individual can become an expression of his inner being. So you see how significantly spiritual science can contribute to the solution of this riddle. But only if you face the whole reality to which the spiritual also belongs, and do not stop merely with the physical reality, can this knowledge be practically applied in life. Therefore only from spiritual science can this knowledge flow in such a way as to benefit the whole of humanity as well as the individual.

Now if we know all that, we can also learn to apply it. Particularly it must be of interest to learn how we can handle the temperaments pedagogically in childhood. For in education the kind of temperament must be carefully observed. With children it is especially important to be able to guide and direct the developing temperament. But it is also important later on for anyone who wishes to train and educate himself to observe what is expressed in his own temperament.

I have pointed out to you here the fundamental types, but naturally in life they do not often appear thus pure. Each person has only the fundamental tone of a temperament, besides which he has something of the others. Napoleon, for example, had in him much of the phlegmatic temperament, although he was a choleric. If we would manage life practically it is important to be able to allow what expresses itself physically to work upon our soul, and give rise to insights about what underlies the physical manifestation.

How important this is we can see best of all if we consider that the temperaments can degenerate, that what may appear to us as one-sidedness can also degenerate. What would the world be without the temperaments — if only one temperament existed for all human beings? The most tiresome place you can imagine! The world would be dreary without the temperaments, not only in the physical, but also in the higher sense. All variety, beauty, and all the richness of life are possible only through the temperaments [. . .]

5. The Bridge Between Universal Spirituality and the Physical

As mentioned previously, we experience the body purely physically through our senses. The mind is an inner psychological experience. However it is not immediately obvious how one works on the other. The Cartesian guillotine dividing body from mind still dominates natural science. We shall see in the following lectures that we can experience the supersensible bodies in the elements of warmth, air, water and solid matter, and thus find ways of bridging this Cartesian split.[1]

Firstly, how can we experience the ego in warmth? We have seen that the ego most clearly manifests in the choleric temperament. The inner enthusiasm that is generated when doing what one really wants to do and working out of one's deepest identity is something that generates inner warmth. Initially this produces soul warmth and later physical warmth as well. Le Shan's advice to cancer patients to 'sing their own song' strengthens their own identity, helping to drive out the alien forces causing cancerous growth.[2] Warmth induced by fever treatment as produced by mistletoe injections, and also very hot baths, helps this struggle against the foreign foe of cancer. When a child develops fever during measles, he or she is not only fractious during the acute phase but also becomes more assertive after the illness has passed, having strengthened his or her identity and personality through the warmth experience.

Secondly, how can we recognize the astral in the air process? Deep emotions invariably have a profound effect on the breathing. We take an inhalatory gasp of astonishment at a surprising experience and breathe out a sigh of relief when all the stress is over. Often asthma attacks are just set off by stress. Very emotionally disturbed children invariably have breathing disturbances. In the author's 21-year experience as a school doctor, their breath is often shallow and quite irregular, being hard to count. One can view flatulence as a certain withdrawal of the astral forces from the etheric and physical in the abdomen. Normally the astral should permeate the etheric and physical in the abdomen as will be seen in the following chapter.

Thirdly, how do we experience the etheric in the fluid system? We may feel drained of energy and weighed down with care if we carry out too much mental work without taking exercise. If in this state we do take exercise it will leave us with a warm glow of energy and well-being, and our step and posture may regain its lightness. This can be seen as stimulation of our heart and circulation, i.e., energizing of the etheric in the fluid organism. There are conditions in which fluid accumulates in the legs (oedema), e.g. in heart failure and terminal cancer. This indicates that the etheric is no longer master of the fluid organism. Some fluid has fallen back into the physical, having lost its lightness (a key feature of the etheric) and become more strongly subject to the influence of gravity. We saw in the last chapter that the sanguine temperament can manifest as a continuous intense stream of immediate thoughts and feeling. These can produce nervousness and insomnia. One way of dealing with this is to use memory images of the events of the day, before going to sleep.

This is best done in reverse sequence. By doing so, the rate of thinking dies down, allowing one to relax and drop off to sleep (well-being is a natural signature of the etheric, as are images 'recollected in tranquillity').

We are commonly aware of an 'upward stream' in us, arising from physical conditions – from food, our hormones, medicine we take, etc. – that influences our mood and sense of well-being. Mainstream medicine is largely concerned with these physical aspects. In the text that follows, though, Steiner refers to the opposite direction of influence: the interaction between moral thoughts stimulating the warmth organism, which in turn produces light in the air organism, then tone in the fluid organism and finally life in the solid organism.

When carrying out a deed for which one is truly motivated, which one does out of the depth of one's being, warm enthusiasm arises as we saw. This in turn radiates joy in feeling life, then works down into a deeper level, producing a sense of well-being (etheric, fluid) and finally makes us healthy in a physical sense.

This stream of forces is well illustrated by those individuals who were able to survive life in a concentration camp. Invariably they had strong religious beliefs. Those who had no such beliefs caved in under a monstrous and inhuman system. Likewise, pensioners who have an active interest in life tend to survive longer than those who just vegetate. Thus through recognizing how the supersensible bodies work in the elements, we can perceive a stream of forces that leads from the ego through the astral and etheric into the physical. This, as Steiner now explains, is the bridge across the Cartesian, mind-body divide.

First 'bridge' lecture: Soul and spirit in man's physical constitution

Today I want to interpolate a theme that may possibly seem to you somewhat remote, but it will be of importance for the further development of subjects we are studying at the present time. We have been able to gather together many details that are essential for a knowledge of man's being. On the one side, we are gradually discovering man's place in the life of the cosmos, and on the other, his place in the life of society. But it will be necessary today to consider certain matters which make for a better understanding of man's being and nature.

When modern scientific thinking is brought to bear on the human being one part only of his being is taken into consideration. No account whatever is taken of the fact that in addition to his physical body, man also has higher members. But we will leave this aside today and think about something that is more or less recognized in science and has also made its way into general consciousness.

In studying the human being, only those elements which can be pictured as solid or solid-fluid are nowadays regarded as belonging to his organism. It is, of course, acknowledged that the fluid and the gaseous elements pass into and out of the human being, but these are not in themselves considered to be integral members of the human organism. The warmth within man which is greater than that of his environment is regarded as a state or condition of his organism, but not as an actual part of his constitution. We shall presently see what I mean by saying this. I have already drawn attention to the fact that when we study the rising and falling of the cerebral fluid through the spinal canal we can observe a regular up-and-down oscillatory movement caused by inhalation and exhalation. When we breathe in, the cerebral fluid is driven upwards and strikes, as it were, against the brain-structure; when we breathe out the fluid sinks again. These processes in the purely liquid components of the human organism are not considered to be part and parcel of the organism itself. The general idea is that man, as a physical structure, consists of the more or less solid, or at most solid-fluid, substances found in him.

Man is pictured as a structure built up from these more or less solid substances [*see diagram*]. The other elements, the fluid element, as I have shown in the example of the cerebral fluid, and the gaseous element, are not regarded by anatomy and physiology as belonging to the human organism as such. It is said, yes, the human being draws in the air which follows certain paths in his body and also has certain definite functions. This air is breathed out again. Then people also speak of the warmth-condition of the body, but in reality they regard the solid element as the only organizing factor and do not realize that in addition to this solid structure they should also see the whole human being as a column of fluid [*blue*], as a being permeated with air [*red*], and as a being in whom there is a definite degree of warmth [*yellow*]. More exact study

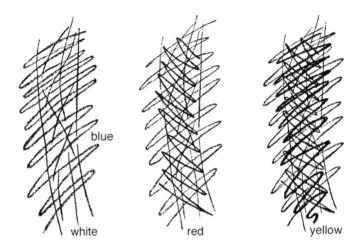

blue

white   red   yellow

shows that just as the solid or solid-fluid constituents are to be considered as an integral part or member of the organism, so the actual fluidity should not be thought of as so much uniform fluid, but as being differentiated and organized — though the process here is a more fluctuating one — and has its own particular significance.

In addition to the solid human being, therefore, we must bear in mind 'fluid man' and also 'gaseous man'. For the air within us, in regard to its organization and its differentiations, is an organism in the same sense as the solid organism, only it is gaseous and in motion. And finally, the warmth in us is not a uniform warmth extending through the whole human being but is also delicately organized. As soon, however, as we begin to speak of the fluid organism, which fills the same space that is occupied by the solid organism, we realize immediately that we cannot speak of this fluid organism in us without speaking of the etheric body, which permeates this fluid organism and fills it with forces. The physical organism exists for itself, as it were; it is the physical body. In so far as we consider it in its entirety, we regard it, to begin with, as a solid organism. This is the physical body.

We then come to consider the fluid organism, which cannot of course be investigated in the same way as the solid organism, by dissection, but which must be conceived as an inwardly mobile, fluid organism. It cannot be studied unless we think of it as permeated by the etheric body.

Thirdly, there is the gaseous organism, which again cannot be studied unless we think of it as permeated with forces by the astral body.

Fourthly, there is the warmth organism with all its inner differentiation. It is permeated by the forces of the ego. That is how we as earthly human beings are constituted today.

1) Solid organism   Physical body
2) Fluid organism   Etheric body
3) Gaseous organism   Astral body
4) Warmth organism   Ego

Let us think, for example, of the blood. Inasmuch as it is mainly fluid, inasmuch as this blood belongs to the fluid organism, we find in the blood the etheric body which permeates it with its forces. But in the blood there is also present what is generally called the warmth condition. But that 'organism' is by no means identical with the organism of the fluid blood as such. If we were to investigate this — and it can also be done with physical methods of investigation — we should find in registering the warmth in the different parts of the human organism that the warmth cannot be identified with the fluid or any other organism.

Directly we reflect about man in this way we feel that it is impossible for our thought to halt within the limits of the human organism itself. We can remain within these limits only if we are thinking merely of the solid organism, which is shut off by the skin from what is outside it. Even this, however, is only apparently so. The solid structure is generally regarded as if it were a firm, self-enclosed block, but it is also inwardly differentiated and is related in manifold ways to the solid earth as a whole. This is obvious from the fact that the different solid substances have, for example, different weights; this alone shows that the solids within the human organism are differentiated, have different specific weights in man. In regard to his physical organism, therefore, the human being is related to the earth as a whole. Nevertheless it is possible, according at least to external evidence, to place spatial limits around the physical organism.

It is different when we come to the second, the fluid organism, which is permeated by the etheric body. This fluid organism cannot be strictly demarcated from the environment. Whatever is fluid in any area of space adjoins the fluid element in its environment. Although the fluid element as such is present in the world outside us in a rarefied state, we cannot make such a definite demarcation between the fluid element within us and the fluid element outside us, as in the case of the solid organism. The boundary between our inner fluid organism and the fluid element in the external world must therefore be left indefinite.

This is even more emphatically the case when we come to consider the gaseous organism, which is permeated by the forces of the astral body. The air within us at any one moment was outside us a moment before, and it will soon be outside again. We are drawing in and giving out the gaseous element all the time. We can really think only of the air as such that surrounds our earth, and say: it penetrates into our organism and withdraws again, but by penetrating into our organism it becomes an integral part of us. In our gaseous organism we actually have something that constantly builds itself up out of the whole atmosphere and then withdraws again into the atmosphere.

Whenever we breathe in, something is built up within us, or, at the very least, each indrawn breath causes a change, a modification, in an upbuilding process within us. Similarly, a destructive, partially destructive process takes place whenever we breathe out. Our gaseous organism undergoes a certain change with every indrawn breath; it is not exactly newly born, but it undergoes a change, both when we breathe in and when we breathe out. When we breathe out, the gaseous organism does not, of course, die; it merely undergoes a change. But there is constant interaction between the gaseous organism within us and the air outside. The usual trivial conceptions of the human organism can only be due to the failure to realize that there is but a slight degree of difference between the gaseous organism and the solid organism.

And now we come to the warmth organism. It is of course quite in keeping with materialistic and mechanistic thought to study only the solid organism and to ignore the fluid organism, the gaseous organism and the warmth organism. But no real knowledge of man's being can be acquired unless we are willing to acknowledge this differentiation into a warmth organism, a gaseous organism, a fluid organism and a physical (solid) earth organism.

The warmth organism is above all the field of the ego. The ego itself is that spiritual organization which imbues with its own forces the warmth within us, and governs and gives it configuration, not only externally but also inwardly. We cannot understand the life and activity of the soul unless we remember that the ego works directly upon the warmth. It is primarily the ego in man which activates the will, generates impulses of will.

How does the ego generate impulses of will? From a different point of view we have spoken of how impulses of will are connected with the earthly sphere, in contrast to the impulses of thought and ideation which are connected with forces outside and beyond the earthly sphere. But how does the ego, which holds together the impulses of will, send these impulses into the organism, into our whole being? This is achieved through the fact that the will works primarily in the warmth organism. An impulse of will proceeding from the ego works upon man's warmth organism. Under present earthly conditions it is not possible for what I shall now describe to you to be there as a concrete reality. Nevertheless it can be envisaged as something that is essentially present in man. It can be envisaged if we disregard the physical organization within the space bounded by the human skin. We disregard this, also the fluid organism, and the gaseous organism. The space then remains filled with nothing but warmth, which is, of course, in communication with the warmth outside. But what is active in this warmth, what sets it in flow, stirs it into movement, makes it into an organism, is the *ego*.

The astral body of man contains within it the forces of feeling. The astral body brings these forces of feeling into physical operation in man's gaseous organism.

As an earthly being, man's constitution is such that, by way of the warmth organism, his ego gives rise to what comes to expression when he acts in the world as a being of will. The feelings experienced in the astral body and coming to expression in the earthly organization manifest as the gaseous organism. And when we come to the etheric organism, to the etheric body, we find within it the *conceptual* process, in so far as this has a pictorial character—more strongly pictorial than we are consciously aware of to begin with, for the physical body still intrudes and tones down the pictures into mental concepts. This process works upon the fluid organism.

This shows us that by taking these different organisms in man into account we come nearer to the life of *soul*. Materialistic observation, which stops short at the solid structure and insists that in the very nature of things water cannot become an organism, is bound to confront the life of soul with complete lack of understanding; for it is precisely in these other organisms that the life of soul comes to immediate expression. The solid organism itself is, in reality, only what provides support for the other organisms. The solid organism stands there as a supporting structure composed of bones, muscles, and so forth. Into this supporting structure is integrated the fluid organism with its own inner differentiation and configuration; in this fluid organism vibrates the etheric body, and within this fluid organism the thoughts are produced. How are the thoughts produced? Through the fact that within the fluid organism something asserts itself in a particular metamorphosis — what we know in the external world as *tone*.

Tone is, in reality, something that leads our ordinary mode of observation very much astray. As earthly human beings we perceive tone as being borne to us by the air. But in point of fact, air is only the transmitter of the tone, which actually weaves in the air. And anyone who assumes that tone in its essence is merely a matter of air vibrations is like someone who says: 'Man has only his physical organism, and there is no soul in it.' If the air vibrations are thought to constitute the essence of the tone, whereas they are in truth merely its external expression, this is the same as seeing only man's physical organism, with no soul in it. The tone which lives in the air is essentially an *etheric* reality. And the tone we hear by way of the air arises through the fact that the air is pervaded by the *tone ether* which is the same as the *chemical ether*.[3] In pervading the air, this chemical ether imparts what lives within it to the air, and we become aware of what we call tone.

This tone ether or chemical ether is essentially active in our fluid organism. We can therefore make the following distinction. In our fluid organism lives our own etheric body; but in addition there penetrates into it (*the fluid organism*) from every direction the tone ether which underlies the tone. Please distinguish carefully here. We have within us our etheric body; it works and is active by giving rise to thoughts in our fluid organism. What may be called the chemical ether continually streams in and out of our fluid organism. Thus we have an etheric organism complete in itself, consisting of chemical ether, warmth ether, light ether, life ether, and in addition we find in it, in a very special sense, the chemical ether which streams in and out by way of the fluid organism.

The astral body, which comes to expression in feeling, operates through the air organism. But still another kind of ether permeating the air is connected especially with the air organism. This is the light ether. Earlier conceptions of the world always emphasized this affinity of the outspreading physical air with the light ether which pervades it. This light ether, which is borne, as it were, by the air and is related to the air even more intimately than tone, also penetrates into our air organism, and it underlies what passes into and out of it. Thus we have our astral body, the bearer of feeling, which is especially active in the air organism and is in constant contact there with the light ether.

And now we come to the ego. This human ego, which by way of the will is active in the warmth organism, is again connected with external warmth, with the instreaming and outstreaming warmth ether [...]

Second 'bridge' lecture: Morality as the source of world creative powers

Yesterday I tried to give certain indications about the human constitution, and at the end it was possible to show that really penetrating study of human nature is able to build a bridge between man's external, physical constitution and what he unfolds in his self-aware inner life. As a rule no such bridge is built, or only very inadequately built, particularly in the science current today. It became clear to us that in order to build this bridge we must know how man's constitution is properly to be regarded. We saw that the solid or solid-fluid organism — which is the sole object of study nowadays and is alone recognized by modern science as organic in the real sense — we saw that this must be regarded as only one of the organisms in man's constitution; that the existence of a fluid organism, a gaseous organism, and a warmth organism must also be recognized. This makes it possible for us also to perceive how those aspects of man's nature penetrate into this delicately organized constitution. Naturally, up to the warmth organism itself, everything is to be conceived as physical body. But it is chiefly the etheric body that takes hold of the fluids within us, of everything that is fluid in the human organism. In everything to do with respiration the astral body is chiefly active, and in the warmth organism the ego works. By recognizing this we can retain our focus on the physical but at the same time also incorporate spiritual realities.

We also studied different levels of consciousness. As I said yesterday, it is usual to take account only of consciousness known to us in waking life from the moment of waking to the moment of falling asleep. We perceive the objects around us, and reason about these perceptions with our intellect; we also have feelings in connection with these perceptions, and we have our impulses of will. But we experience this whole nexus of consciousness as something which, in its qualities, differs completely from the physical which alone is taken account of by ordinary science. It is not possible, without further ado, to build a bridge from these imponderable, incorporeal experiences in the domain of consciousness to the other objects of perception studied in physiology or physical anatomy. But in regard to consciousness too, we know from ordinary life that in addition to waking consciousness there is dream consciousness, and we heard yesterday that dreams are essentially pictures or symbols of inner organic processes. Something is going on within us all the time, and in our dreams it comes to expression in pictures. I said that we may dream of coiling snakes when we have some intestinal disorder, or we may dream of an excessively hot stove and wake up with palpitations of the heart. The overheated stove symbolized an irregular beating of the heart, the snakes symbolized the intestines, and so forth. Dreams point us to our organism; the consciousness of dreamless sleep is, as it were, an experience of nullity, of the void. But I explained that this experience of the void is necessary in order for us to feel ourselves connected with our bodily nature. As an ego we would feel no connection with our body if we did not leave it during sleep and seek for it again on waking. It is through the deprivation undergone between falling asleep and waking that we are able to feel ourselves united with the body.

So from the ordinary consciousness, which has really nothing to do with our own essential being beyond the fact that it enables us to have perceptions and ideas, we are led to dream consciousness which has to do with actual bodily processes. We are therefore led to the body. And we are led to the body even more strongly when we pass into the consciousness of dreamless sleep. Thus we can say that on the one hand our conception of the life of soul is such that it leads us to the body. And our conception of the bodily constitution, comprising as it does the fluid organism, the gaseous organism, the warmth organism and thus becoming by degrees more rarefied, leads us to the realm of soul. It is absolutely necessary to take these things into consideration if we are to reach a view of the world that can really satisfy us.

The great question with which we have been concerning ourselves for weeks, the cardinal question in man's conception of the world, is this: how is the moral world order connected with the physical world order? As has been said so often, the prevailing world view — which relies entirely upon natural science for knowledge of the outer physical world and can only resort to previous religious beliefs when it is a matter of any really comprehensive understanding of the life of soul, for in modern psychology there is no longer any such understanding — this world view is unable to build a bridge. There, on the one hand, is the physical world. According to the modern world view, this is a conglomeration formed from a primeval nebula, and everything will eventually become a kind of slagheap in the universe. This is the picture of the evolutionary process presented to us by the science of today, and it is the one and only picture in which a really honest modern scientist can find reality.

Within this picture a moral world order has no place. It is there on its own. Man receives the moral impulses into himself as impulses of soul. But if the assertions of natural science are true, everything that is astir with life, and finally man himself, came out of the primeval nebula; and moral ideals simply well up in him. And when, as is alleged, the world finally becomes a slagheap, this will also be the graveyard of all moral ideals. They will have vanished. No bridge can possibly be built, and what is worse, modern science cannot, without being inconsistent, admit the existence of morality in its world order. Only if modern science is inconsistent can it accept a moral dimension as valid. It cannot do so if it is consistent. The root of all this is that the only kind of anatomy in existence is concerned exclusively with the solid organism, and no account is taken of the fact that man also has within him a fluid organism, a gaseous organism, and a warmth organism. Picture to yourselves that as well as the solid organism with its configuration of bones, muscles, nerve fibres, and so forth, you also have a fluid organism and a gaseous organism—though these are of course fluctuating and inwardly mobile—and a warmth organism. If you picture this you will more easily understand what I shall now have to say on the basis of spiritual-scientific observation.

Think of someone whose very soul is fired with enthusiasm for a high moral ideal, for the ideal of generosity, freedom, goodness, love, or whatever it may be. He may also feel enthusiasm for examples of the practical expression of these ideals. But nobody can conceive that the enthusiasm which fires the soul penetrates into the bones and muscles as they are described by modern physiology or anatomy. If you really reflect carefully, however, you will find it quite possible to conceive that when someone has enthusiasm for a high moral ideal, this enthusiasm has an effect upon the warmth organism. There, you see, we have come from the realm of soul into the physical!

Taking this as an example, we may say that moral ideals come to expression in an enhancement of warmth in the warmth organism. Not only is man warmed in soul through what he experiences in the way of moral ideals, but he becomes organically warmer as well—though this is not so easy to prove with physical instruments. Moral ideals, then, have a stimulating, invigorating effect upon the warmth organism.

You must think of this as a real and concrete occurrence: enthusiasm for a moral ideal—stimulation of the warmth organism. There is more vigorous activity in the warmth organism when the soul is fired by a moral ideal. Neither does this remain without effect upon the rest of our constitution. As well as the warmth organism we also have the air organism. We inhale and exhale the air; but during this inbreathing and outbreathing process the air is within us. It is of course inwardly in movement, in fluctuation, but in the same way as the warmth organism it is an actual air organism in man. Warmth, quickened by a moral ideal, works in turn upon the air organism, because warmth pervades the whole human organism, pervades every part of it. The effect upon the air organism is not that of warming only, for when the warmth, stimulated in the warmth organism, works upon the air organism, it imparts to it something that I can only call a *source of light.* Sources of light, as it were, are imparted to the air organism, so that moral ideals which have a stimulating effect upon the warmth organism produce sources of light in the air organism. To external perception and for ordinary consciousness these sources of light are not in themselves luminous, but they manifest in man's astral body. To begin with, they are curbed—if I may use this expression—through the air that is within us. They are, so to speak, still dark light, in the sense that the seed of the plant is not yet a developed plant. Nevertheless man has a source of light within him through the fact that he can be fired with enthusiasm for moral ideals, for moral impulses.

We also have within us the fluid organism. Warmth, stimulated in the warmth organism by moral ideals, produces in the air organism what may be called a source of light which remains, to begin with, curbed and hidden. Within the fluid organism—because everything in man's constitution interpenetrates—a process takes place which I said yesterday actually underlies tone externally conveyed in the air. I said that the air is only the body of the tone, and anyone who regards the essential reality of tone as a matter of vibrations of the air speaks of tones just as he would speak of man as having nothing except the outwardly visible physical body. The air with its vibrating waves is nothing but the outer body of the tone. In the human being this tone, this *spiritual tone,* is not produced in the air organism through a moral ideal, but in the fluid organism. The sources of tone therefore arise in the fluid organism.

We regard the solid organism as the densest of all, as the one that supports and bears all the others. Within it, too, something is produced as in the case of the other organisms. In the solid organism there is produced what we call a *seed of life*. But it is an etheric not a physical seed of life such as issues from the female organism at a birth. This etheric seed, which lies in the deepest levels of subconsciousness, is actually the primal source of tone and, in a certain sense, even the source of light. This is entirely hidden from ordinary consciousness but it is there within the human being.

Think of all the experiences in your life that aspiration to moral ideas has given rise to — be it that they attracted you merely as ideas, or that you saw them coming to expression in others, or that you felt inwardly satisfied by having put such impulses into practice, by letting your deeds be fired by moral ideals. All this goes down into the air organism as a source of light, into the fluid organism as a source of tone, into the solid organism as a source of life.

These processes are withdrawn from the field of man's consciousness but they operate within him nevertheless! They are released when he lays aside his physical body at death. What is thus produced in us through moral ideals, or through the loftiest and purest ideas, does nor bear immediate fruit during the life between birth and death. Moral ideas as such become fruitful only in so far as we remain in the life of ideas, and in so far as we feel a certain satisfaction in moral deeds performed. But this is a matter merely of memory, and has nothing to do with what actually penetrates down into our different organisms as the result of enthusiasm for moral ideals.

So we see that our whole constitution, beginning with the warmth organism, is actually permeated by moral ideals. And when at death the etheric body, the astral body and the ego emerge from the physical body, these higher members of our human nature are filled with all the impressions we have had. Our ego was living in the warmth organism when it was quickened by moral ideas. We were living in an air organism, into which were implanted sources of *light* which now, after death, go forth into the cosmos together with us. In our fluid organism, *tone* was kindled which now becomes part of the music of the spheres, resounding from us into the cosmos. And we bring *life* with us when we pass out into the cosmos through the portal of death.

You will now begin to have an inkling of what the life that pervades the universe really is. Where are the sources of life? They lie in what quickens those moral ideals which fire man with enthusiasm. We come to the point of saying to ourselves that if today we allow ourselves to be inspired by moral ideals, these will carry forth life, tone and light into the universe and will become *world-creative.* We carry out into the universe world-creative power, and the source of this power is the moral element.

So when we study the *whole* human being we find a bridge between moral ideals and what works as life-giving force in the physical world, even in the chemical sense. For tone works in the chemical sense by assembling substances and dispersing them again. Light in the world has its source in moral stimuli, in the warmth organisms of human beings. Thus we look into the future — new worlds take shape. And as in the case of the plant we must go back to the seed, so in the case of these future worlds that will come into being we must go back to the seeds that lie in us as moral ideals.

And now think of theoretical ideas in contrast to moral ideals. In the case of theoretical ideas, everything is different. No matter how significant these ideas may be, theoretical ideas produce the very opposite effect to that of stimulus. They *cool down* the warmth organism — that is the difference.

Moral ideas, or ideas of a moral-religious character, which fire us with enthusiasm and become impulses for deeds, work as world-creative powers. Theoretical ideas and speculations have a cooling, subduing effect upon the warmth organism. Because this is so, they also have a *paralysing* effect upon the air organism and upon the source of light within it; they have a *deadening* effect upon tone, and an *extinguishing* effect upon life. In our theoretical ideas the creations of the pre-existing world come to their end. When we formulate theoretical ideas a universe dies in them. Thus do we bear within us the death of a universe and the dawn of a universe.

Here we come to the point where he who is initiated into the secrets of the universe cannot speak as so many speak today, of the conservation of energy or the conservation of matter.[4] It is simply not true that matter is conserved for ever. Matter dies to the point of nullity, to a zero point. In our own organism, energy dies to the point of nullity through the fact that we formulate theoretical thoughts. But if we did not do so, if the universe did not continually die in us, we should not be human in the true sense. Because the universe dies in us, we are endowed with self-awareness and are able to think about the universe. But these thoughts are the corpse of the universe. We become conscious of the universe as a corpse only, and it is this that makes us man.

A past world dies within us, down to its very matter and energy. It is only because a new universe at once begins to dawn that we do not notice this dying of matter and its immediate rebirth. Through man's theoretical thinking, matter — substantiality — is brought to its end; through his *moral* thinking matter and cosmic energy are imbued with new life. Thus what goes on inside the boundary of the human skin is connected with the dying and birth of worlds. This is how the moral order and the natural order are connected. The natural world dies away in man; in the realm of the moral a new natural world comes to birth.

Moral ideals
stimulate the warmth organism
produce sources of light in the air organism
produce sources of tone in the fluid organism
produce sources of life in the solid organism

Theoretical thoughts
cool down the warmth organism
paralyse the sources of light
deaden the sources of tone
extinguish life

Because of unwillingness to consider these things, ideas of the imperishability of matter and energy were invented. If energy and matter were imperishable there would be no moral world order. But today people desire to keep this truth concealed and modern thought has every reason to do so, because otherwise it would have to eliminate the moral world order — which in actual fact it does by speaking of the law of the conservation of matter and energy. If matter is conserved or energy is conserved, the moral world order is nothing but an illusion, a mirage. We can understand world evolution only if we grasp how, out of this 'illusory' moral world-order — for so it is when grasped in thoughts — new worlds come into being.

Nothing of this can be grasped if we study only the solid component of man's constitution. To understand it we must pass from the solid organism through the fluid and gaseous organisms to the warmth organism. Man's connection with the universe can be understood only if the physical is traced upwards to that rarefied state wherein the soul can be directly active in the rarefied physical element, as for example in warmth. Then it is possible to find the connection between body and soul.

However many treatises on psychology may be written,

if they are based on what is studied today in anatomy and physiology it will not be possible to find any transition to the life of soul from this solid or solid-fluid bodily constitution. The life of soul will not be revealed as such. But if we trace our bodily substance back to warmth, a bridge can be built from what exists in the body as warmth to what works out of the soul into the warmth in the human organism. There is warmth both outside and within the human organism. As we have heard, in man's constitution warmth is an organism; the soul and spirit take hold of this warmth organism, and by way of warmth everything comes to expression that we experience as moral thought and act. I do not of course mean morality in a narrow sense, but in its totality — that is to say, all those impulses that come to us, for instance, when we contemplate the majesty of the universe, when we say to ourselves, 'We are born out of the cosmos and we are responsible for what goes on in the world — those impulses that come to us when the knowledge yielded by spiritual science inspires us to work for the sake of the future.

When we regard spiritual science itself as a source of what is moral, this more than anything else can fill us with enthusiasm for the moral. And this enthusiasm, born of spiritual-scientific knowledge, becomes in itself a source of morality in the higher, wider sense. But what is generally called 'moral' represents no more than a subordinate sphere of a more universal sense of morality.

All the ideas we evolve about the external world, about nature in her finished array, are theoretical ideas. No matter with what exactitude we envisage a machine in terms of mathematics and the principles of mechanics, or the universe in the sense of the Copernican system, this is nothing but theoretical thinking and the ideas thus formulated constitute a force of death within us — a corpse of the universe within us.

These matters create deeper and deeper insight into the universe in its totality. There are two orders, a natural order and a moral order in juxtaposition, but the two are one. This is a truth that we need to realize today. Otherwise we must ever and again be asking ourselves how our moral impulses take effect in a world in which a natural order alone prevails. This indeed was the terrible problem that weighed upon people in the nineteenth century and early twentieth century: how is it possible to conceive of any transition from the natural world into the moral world, from the moral world into the natural world?

The fact is that nothing can help to solve this perplexing, fateful problem except spiritual-scientific insight into both nature, on the one hand, and spirit on the other [...]

6. The Constellation of the Supersensible Bodies

The following lecture is another essential key to Steiner's insights into the human being. In it Steiner describes how each supersensible body works in a different way in head, metabolic and limb system and thoracic system – distinctions necessary to avoid much confusion. It is helpful to read this lecture in conjunction with the more complex second medical course given on 11 April 1921,[1] as it deals with related themes.

The illustration on p. 125 shows in diagrammatic form the different roles played by the supersensible bodies in each of the three main areas of the human physical body – head, chest and limbs/metabolism.

Steiner describes the 'I' or ego as living 'outside us' in sense perception. How can we understand this? Something of an ego force issues from our eyes in the glance, for instance, and is sent out to the objects we perceive, uniting with them and bringing them back to us impressions. There is certainly nothing physical about this. The etheric forces, too, which originally form and build up the physical, become to some extent free of the body in abstract thinking. When creating images in our mind – a triangle or circle for instance – we can experience an inner thought space, giving us a certain separation from the world outside, and allowing us to create a rich inner world. In our heads we are capable of being wide awake, and this occurs where the supersensible bodies are at least partially liberated from immersion in the physical body.

In the metabolic and limb system, in contrast, we are usually deeply unconscious and unaware of the processes unfolding there. Here strong forces use the digestive juices (astral) to break down and destroy the food we absorb. Our digestive system is also the anabolic centre and close to the reproductive system (strong etheric forces). All these forces work in a bodily or somatic fashion, rather than being freed as consciousness, as they are in the head. The ego, however, is still to some extent body-free in the metabolic sphere, though it unites with the body in movement and willed actions.

In the thorax or middle system of the human being, a mediating state of consciousness holds sway, and it is here that our feeling life is based. Feeling is equivalent in some ways to dreaming. In the to and fro of our feelings, with their antipathy and sympathy, the astral has a looser connection with the body than it does in metabolism, but still a more intimate connection with physical processes than in clear thinking. The middle system, according to Steiner, is also the source of our health, mediating between the opposite poles of thinking and will. When we wish to recover from too much headwork or physical exertion, we often like to bathe in our feelings and be refreshed by going to an artistic performance of some kind – a play or concert perhaps. This can rejuvenate us bodily as well as emotionally through the action of the etheric body, as is also borne out by the practice of artistic therapies such as painting, sculpture, music and eurythmy.

Now we must come back again to these things, in a different way. For instance, we must become clear that we human beings, with our ego, are distinct from all the animals. Our ego, you know, is still very much asleep in the great majority of people. If one thinks the ego is very wide awake, then one is in error. For in the will, as I have already explained, man is really asleep, and inasmuch as the ego busies itself in will, we have to do not with something that confronts us as ego, but with something that really stands before us as the night does. You see, we reckon with night, too—do we not—in our life, although the night is dark. For life does not only consist of what is clear as day, but it consists also of the nights. But in a way they are always struck out of the course of time in our awareness. It is the same with our ego. Our ego, for ordinary consciousness, is really characterized by the fact of it not being there. It is certainly there, but not for consciousness. One misses something there, and therefore one sees the ego. It is really as if there was a white wall, and one place has not been covered with white, so there one sees the black. And so in ordinary consciousness one really sees the ego as what is extinguished. And it is so, too, during waking. The ego is really always asleep, but as a sleeping being it appears through thoughts, feelings and ideas, and thus it is perceived even in ordinary consciousness—that means, we believe we perceive it. We can say, therefore, that our ego is not really perceived directly.

Now a prejudiced psychology, a prejudiced theory of the soul, believes that this ego really lies within us—where our muscles, flesh, bones, etc., are, there is the ego also. If one were to give but a superficial glance at life one would very quickly know that this is not so. But it is difficult to bring such deliberations before people today. I tried to do it in 1910 in my lecture at the Philosophical Congress in Bologna. But so far no one has understood this lecture. I tried there to show the real state of affairs regarding the ego. This ego really lies in each perception, it actually lies in all that makes an impression upon us. Not inside in my flesh and bones does the ego lie, but in what I can perceive with my eyes. When you see red anywhere—in a flower, perhaps—you cannot separate the red impression from the flower itself. The ego is concerned in all this. The ego is in fact bound up with your soul content. But your soul content is certainly not in your bones, you spread it throughout all space. Thus the ego is within you still less than the air you inhale, still less than the air which was in you a short time ago. This ego is bound up with each perception and with all that is basically, actually, outside you. It is only active within because it sends into you the forces from your perceptions. And, furthermore, the ego is connected with something else as well. You only need to walk—in other words to unfold your will. There at any rate your ego walks with you, or takes part in the movement, and whether you run, whether you skip or anything else, whether you turn round and round, whether you dance or jump, the ego goes through it all with you. In everything which arises in you as movement the ego enters too. But this, as you know, is not strictly within you, it takes you with it. If you dance a round dance, do you think the dance is within you? It would certainly have no room in you. How would it have room? But the ego is there, too. The ego goes through the dance, too. So in your perceptions, in your actions, there lies the ego. But that is not being really within you in the full sense of word, as your stomach is within you; there is always something of this ego which is fundamentally outside you. It is just as much outside the head as it is outside the legs, only that in walking it takes a great share in the movements that the legs make. The ego really participates very much in the movements made by the legs, but participates less in the [*physical*] activity of the head.

But what is it through which the legs or the limbs in general, together with the metabolic system, are distinguished from the head? You see, in the head, the etheric body and the astral body, too, are relatively independent. The head is most of all physical body. The head, which is such an old fellow already, since it originates from our previous incarnation, has become most physical of all—it is really the oldest earth inhabitant. In the legs or limb system and metabolism, in contrast, the etheric body and the astral body are inwardly bound up with the physical body. Only the ego is relatively free from the legs and only takes the legs with it when they move. And it is the same with the metabolic system. The metabolic organs are essentially bound up with the etheric and the astral body. So we can ask what it is that distinguishes the human head from our metabolic and limb system? It is the fact that the head has actually a free etheric body, free astral body and free ego. Our limb and metabolic system has only a relatively free ego, while the etheric body and astral body are bound up with the physical body. They are not free from it.

Now perhaps the matter will be still clearer to you if I put the following before you. Suppose that one day it occurred to your astral body or your etheric body – to the part of it that has to look after your metabolic and limb system – to behave in the same way as the etheric body and astral body of the head. Imagine that it had the distinct idea that it would be free too. Let us say, for example, that the astral body of your metabolic being wanted to behave as its 'colleague', the astral body of the head, is allowed to behave. It is only another portion of the astral body, so I say 'its colleague'. What happens then? Something happens which ought not to happen at all, because it contradicts the laws of the human form. What happens is that our 'lower man' wants to become a head, that it wants to become like the head. And the peculiarity is that the same thing that is healthy in the case of the head makes the 'lower man' ill. Fundamentally, it is a general characteristic of all illnesses of the lower part of the body that the body takes on the configuration of the head.

It was only a special instance of this that I explained, for instance, regarding cancer, in a lecture in Stuttgart or Zurich. There I pointed out that cancer formation is due to the fact that in a part of the human body where there should be no internal sense organs formed the astral body suddenly begins to want to form sense organs there, to wake up and perceive things. The cancer is only something wishing to be ear or eye in a wrong place. It grows inside. It wants to form an ear or eye there. When therefore the astral body or the etheric body of the lower body desires to act as the astral body or etheric body in the head act, then disease begins in the lower body.

And, likewise, if the head also begins—and this occurs to a slight extent in a migraine-type condition—to want to live like the lower body so that it draws its astral body or its etheric body into its activity, then the head becomes ill. When it draws its etheric body in, migraine conditions ensue; where it draws its astral body inside, still worse things arise.

These are facts which show you how complicated our human nature is. One cannot study human nature in the shallow ways that modern science does, but one must study it so that one observes it in all its complexity and sees that the head cannot be like the lower body—it can only become ill if it does so. When, therefore, the cerebrum begins to develop its metabolism too strongly, illness ensues. And these excessive secretion processes come about if the head is encroaching too strongly on its etheric body. As soon, however, as our lower body is left to itself, that is to say, becomes headlike, acquires a kind of disposition to develop sense organs, then its diseases develop. You can say, therefore, that the head of man has a free astral body, free etheric, free ego. Our metabolic-limb nature has a dependent etheric body, that is to say dependent on the physical material, dependent astral body and only a free ego. And our 'middle region', rhythmic man, has a dependent etheric body, free astral body and free ego.

Head — free etheric, free astral, free ego
Rhythmic man — dependent etheric, free astral, free ego
Metabolic-limb man — dependent etheric, dependent astral, free ego

Here you have a survey of the human constitution from an aspect that is extraordinarily important, because by this means you get an impression of how the ego has freedom in respect to us, how the ego really — that is to say, from waking to falling asleep — works into the human being, how it is really bound up with external perception and with what man makes as external movements, but how it does not really penetrate fully into the human body [. . .]

7. The Invisible Human Within Us: The Pathology Underlying Therapy

The following lecture is a key one in understanding the essence of anthroposophical medicine, and gives insight into many medical phenomena. Oddly enough, it was not given to doctors.

The idea of the invisible human within us is very helpful in understanding the mind-body relationship. We saw in the last lecture that the supersensible bodies (etheric, astral and ego) work very strongly into the physical in the metabolic-limb system, whereas in the head they are somewhat withdrawn, allowing waking consciousness to unfold. In the lecture which follows we find that the ego in the metabolic-limb system is so to say clothed with these supersensible bodies working in the blood. In the head, the centre of the nervous and sense system, in contrast, the ego works in a naked, direct way. In the metabolic system the ego works in an anabolic (synthesizing) way, whereas in the head it works in a catabolic (breaking down) way. We already saw that exercise can give us a sense of well-being, whereas headwork can make us tense and nervous. In this lecture Steiner examines these tendencies at the point they become pathological. One such tendency was also illustrated in the work of Le Shan,[1] who describes the cancer patient as typically someone who complies with outer demands and is not sure what he wishes to gain from life. In such a person outer forces and impressions dominate. Le Shan's psychotherapeutic method involves getting the patient to discover what he really wants from life and then realize this actively (will).

Where, in such a case, the upper supersensible bodies (ego and astral) do not work strongly into the etheric and physical, the subject tends to be lanky and pale, since etheric forces have been unchecked from above in their upward growth. This is also a typical picture of the melancholic temperament (see chapter 4). The choleric person, in contrast, tends to be small in stature (e.g. Napoleon), for here the upper supersensible bodies (ego and astral) have worked down forcefully upon the etheric, inhibiting its upward growth to produce a stocky build.

This lecture also helps us gain insight into the alchemical view of pathology in which head dominance produces degenerative, hardening illnesses (sal) while metabolic-limb dominance produces inflammatory, dissolving diseases (sulphur). When these two forces are in balance, heart and lung forces are well developed and health (mercury) will ensue.

A schematic summary at the end of the lecture helps provide an overview of the opposite poles Steiner is referring to here, between the 'invisible human being' forces and those of conscious ego activity.

When we consider the human being, two entities can be clearly distinguished. You will recall that in various recent studies I explained how the human being's physical organization is spiritually prepared during pre-earthly life. In a certain sense it is then sent down as spiritual organization before the human being enters with his ego into earthly existence. This spiritual organization continues to be active essentially during the entire physical life on earth, but it does not express itself during physical earthly life as something outwardly visible. The outwardly visible aspect of this spiritual organization is essentially cast off at birth, consisting of the embryonic membranes that envelop the human embryo during its development—the chorion, the allantois, the amnion, the yolk sac—everything, in other words, that is cast away as physical organization when the human being attains a free physical existence on leaving the maternal body. Yet this pre-earthly organization continues to be active in the human being throughout his entire life. It is somewhat different in character, however, from the body-soul-spirit activity of the human being during his physical earthly life. And this is what I would like to speak about today.

In a certain sense, then, we have an invisible human being within us. It is contained in our growth-forces, as well as in those hidden forces through which nourishment occurs. It is contained in everything in which the human being is not consciously active. Its work extends into this unconscious activity, right into growth activity, into the daily restoration of forces through nutrition. And this work is the after-effect of pre-earthly existence, which in earthly existence becomes a body of forces that is active in us but does not come to conscious manifestation. To begin with I would like to describe to you the character of this invisible human being, which we all carry within us, contained in our forces of growth and nutrition, as well as in our reproductive forces.

Proceeding schematically, we can say that this invisible human also contains the ego, the astral organization, the etheric organization (and therefore the body of formative forces), and the physical organization. Of course, in the human being after birth the physical organization of this invisible being is contained within the rest of the human physical organization, but in the course of today's considerations you will begin to understand how this invisible entity can take hold of the physical organization.

Drawn schematically it would look like this [*see drawing*].

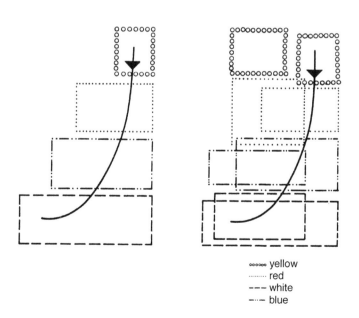

ooooo yellow
········· red
--- white
-··- blue

In this invisible being we have first the ego organization [*yellow*]; then we have the astral organization [red], then the etheric organization [*blue*], and finally we have the physical organization [*white*]. This physical organization of the invisible human being within us penetrates only into nutrition and growth processes, into everything where the lower being, as we have often described it—the metabolic-limb being—manifests in the human organization. All currents, all effects of forces in this invisible human being proceed from the ego organization into the astral, then into the etheric, and on into the physical organization [*see arrow*]. They then spread out in the physical organization. In the human embryo, what we call here the physical organization of the invisible human being is present in the embryonic envelopes, in the embryonic sheaths, the chorion, the allantois, the amnion, and the yolk sac and so forth. In the human being after birth, however, what is here called the physical organization is contained in nourishing and restorative processes in the human being. Thus, outwardly, this physical organization is not separated from the remaining physical organization of the human being but is united with it.

In a certain sense, then, in addition to this invisible human being we have the visible human being which we encounter after birth. I will sketch this visible human being right next to the invisible one [*see drawing*]. This is how the mutual interpenetration of the physical and superphysical human being would appear during earthly life. During earthly life there is a continuous stream from ego to astral body, to etheric body, to physical body [*see arrows*]. In the human being after birth, this stream flows into the metabolic-limb organization, in the forces of our outer movement, and also in the forces of inner movement that carry ingested food into the entire organization up to the brain.

In addition to this, however, there is a direct intervention of forces that enter the entire human being directly from the ego [*see drawing 1*]. An activity thus penetrates us,

ooooo yellow
········· red
——— white
—··— blue
—▴— green

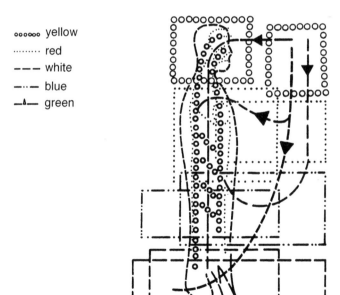

1

a stream that flows directly from the ego into the nerve-sense organization without first passing through the astral body and etheric body; instead this stream lays hold of man's physical body directly. Naturally this penetration is strongest in the head, where most of the sense organs are concentrated, but I should actually draw this stream in such a way that it spreads out via the skin-senses, over the entire human being, just as I would have to draw a stream for the taking in of food through the mouth. Schematically, however, my drawing is quite correct. In the human head, then, we have one organization that flows up from below, proceeding from the ego but passing through the astral, etheric and physical and then up to the ego. We have another stream that enters the physical directly and flows downwards.

If we examine the human organism, we arrive at the insight that this unmediated stream, which enters the physical directly from the ego and then branches out over the whole body, proceeds along the nerve pathways [*see drawing 1, yellow*]. Thus when the human nerves spread out in the organism, the outwardly visible nerve-strand is the visible sign of these outspreading streams that enter the entire organism directly from the ego, proceeding from the ego into the physical organization without mediation. The ego organization at first runs along the pathways of the nerves. This has an essentially destructive effect on the organism. There the spirit enters directly into physical matter, and wherever the spirit enters physical matter directly a destructive process occurs, so that along the nerve pathways, proceeding from the senses, a delicate death process spreads out through the human organism.

The other stream, which in the invisible human being goes through the astral, etheric and physical bodies, can be traced in us by following the blood pathways up to the senses [*see drawing 1, red*]. Thus when we examine man as we encounter him here on earth, we can say that the ego flows in the blood. But the ego flows in such a way that it first ensouls its forces through the astral organization and through the etheric and physical organizations. After first taking along the astral and etheric organizations, the ego streams through the physical organization in the blood from below upwards. Thus the entire invisible human being flows in the blood as a constructive process, as a growth process, as the process that constantly renews us by working through our food. This stream flows in the human being from below upwards (speaking schematically), pours itself into the senses, and therefore also into the skin, and encounters the other stream which, from the ego, takes hold of the physical organization directly. Actually, however, this whole matter is even more complex, because we must also consider the breathing process.

In the breathing process, the ego flows into the astral body, but then it goes directly into the lungs with help of the air. Thus something from the supersensible human being also underlies the breathing process, but not in the same way as occurs in the nerve-sense process, where the ego takes hold of the physical organization directly. In the breathing process, the ego permeates itself with the astral forces, taking hold of oxygen; and only then, no longer as pure ego organization but as ego-astral organization, does it take hold of the organism with the help of the breathing process [*see drawing 1, third arrow*]. It could also be said that the breathing process is a weakened process of destruction, a weakened death process. The actual death process is the nerve-sense process, while the breathing process is a weakened breaking-down process.

This is countered by the process in which the ego further strengthens itself by streaming up to the etheric body and only then is taken up [*see drawing 1, fourth arrow*]. This process, taking place mainly in the supersensible so that it cannot be traced by normal physiology, is active in the pulse, where it is still outwardly perceptible. It is a restorative process, not as strong as the direct metabolic-restorative process, but rather a weakened restorative process. And this then encounters the breathing process.

The breathing process is to a certain extent a destructive process. Our life would be much shorter if we absorbed more oxygen. The more the process of carbon dioxide formation in the blood counters the absorption of oxygen in the breathing process, the longer our life will be.

Thus everything interacts within the organism. And in order really to understand what is going on, one needs to understand the supersensible human being, because its outwardly visible aspects were cast off with the embryonic membranes and are active in the human being after birth only in the form of invisible forces. These forces can be clearly delineated, however, if we proceed from anthroposophical understanding of the human being.

If, for example, we examine the eye with this anthroposophical understanding, we see that the blood process courses through the eye in fine ramifications [*see drawing 2, red*]. This is taken hold of by the nerve process (yellow), going in the opposite direction. The blood process always moves towards the periphery in the human being, moving centrifugally; the nerve process, which is in fact a breaking down process, is always directed centripetally, towards our interior. All processes that occur in the human being are metamorphoses of these two processes.

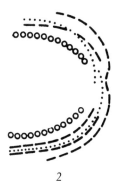

2

When the dynamics between pulse and breathing are properly balanced, then the lower human being is properly connected to the upper. If this is the case and no external injuries intervene, an individual should be basically healthy. Only when breaking down processes predominate will these encroach on activities in the organism. The human being becomes ill because something foreign accumulates in his organism that has not been worked through in the right way, that is, something containing excess destructive forces, containing too much that is akin to outer physical nature surrounding the human being on earth.

The spiritual element's direct penetration of the organism by way of the ego brings about all those alien formation processes of a pathological nature. These alien formations may not manifest immediately in physical symptoms, but could manifest in the fluid and even in the airy aspect of the human being, but they are still alien formations. They can develop, and if they are not countered by a healing process that flows from below along the pathways of the blood, they cannot dissolve. These formations have the tendency to form tumour-like accumulations in the body and then to fragment within. If the blood-formation process counters them in the right way, they can dissolve and again become part of the general life of the body. But when an excessive breakdown process from above downwards causes an obstruction, the catabolic (destructive) process takes hold of one of the organs. Foreign bodies are then formed, which are first exudative, tumour-like, but then have the tendency to run their course like the external processes of earthly nature and fall to pieces. In this case we need to understand that not enough of the supersensible human being is taken up along the path I have drawn here next to the physical human being.

You see, one cannot speak directly about healing through human skill, because the moment that too much activity is developed in relation to the nerve-sense organization, in a centripetal direction—i.e., when too many outer environment-type processes are 'stuffed' into the human being so that these tumour-like formations develop somewhere, which then fall to pieces—in that moment the other system, which runs along the blood vessels, becomes rebellious. It wants to bring about healing, wants to penetrate the organism with the proper astral and etheric forces that can come from below. It wants to prevent the ego, or the ego working with the astral body, from acting alone. Such a revolutionary principle in the human organism has to be assumed by the healer, and healing consists of supporting, by external means, what is already present in the organism as an original healing force.

When a tumour-like formation arises, it is a symptom that ego activity is not penetrating in the right way out of the etheric body. Ego activity does assert itself, but may at times be unable to get access to the tumour. We might then support the etheric body in this direction so that it can become effective. It can become active in the right way if it is first permeated by the ego and astral body and then becomes active. What comes from above and has not taken up etheric activity, but at most ego and astral activity, poisons the organism. When the etheric body confronts this, when we counter the ego and astral activity with etheric activity, we support the healing process already present and striving to be active in the human organization. We only really have to know, in such a case, what remedies are needed for the etheric organization, permeated in the right way by astral and ego organization, to take hold of the body. In other words, in such a case we simply need to strengthen the etheric organization with a remedy. Therefore we must know which remedy will make the etheric organization stronger in such a case, so that it can use its constructive force to counter an excessive destructive force. Thus we can see that we will never comprehend the pathology that underlies therapy unless we take into account the invisible human being.

It may also happen, however, that when a person is born he does not penetrate strongly enough with his ego and astral organization—with his soul-spiritual organization—into the physical organization. The soul-spiritual organization does not push its way into the physical organization sufficiently. Then in this individual there will continually be a preponderance of the growth forces active from below upwards, which do not acquire sufficient weight through integration of the physical organization. An individual can be born in such a way that the invisible human being takes insufficient hold of his physical body, refusing to penetrate into the blood process in the right way. Then man's spirit cannot approach the blood process. In such individuals we can see the consequences of this from childhood on. They remain pale and thin or, because of the predominating growth forces, rapidly shoot up. Then the soul-spiritual element cannot properly enter the organism. And because the body refuses to take up the soul-spiritual, our goal must be to weaken the overly strong etheric body whose activity has become too dominant. In such pale, lanky individuals we must strive to contain the hypertrophic, overly strong activity in the etheric body, restraining it to a proper degree. By this means we can bring weight into the body; the blood, for example, by receiving the necessary iron content, receives the appropriate heaviness. Thus the etheric body ceases to be so active in an upward direction, and its effect on the upper human being is weakened.

In such individuals another condition might be noticed: what I would like to call the night processes predominate over the day processes. You could say that at night the physical-etheric organization of every normal person refuses to assimilate the soul-spiritual. This night organization of a person lying in bed — not of the invisible human being who is outside it — is too strong in those people who have a sort of inborn consumption, as I have just described. In such cases, the day organization must be supported and strengthened. This means that it has to be given a certain weight by encouraging the breaking down or catabolic processes. If one enhances the breaking down processes and inwardly there arises a hardening, ultimately fragmenting process (in healing, of course, this must happen only to a small extent) then the over-exuberant force of the etheric body is restrained and the tendency towards consumption is held back.

In this way, through knowledge of the entire human being, we can comprehend the curious interaction between health and disease. This interaction is always present and is essentially balanced by what occurs between pulse and breath. If we then come to know by what outer means one or the other can be enhanced, it will be possible to support the natural healing processes that are always present, but, I would say, not always able to arise. Then a totally foreign process cannot be introduced into the human organism. There is something continually taking place within the human organism. When some kind of alien process is introduced, it is at once transformed into its opposite within the organism. If you eat something, the food contains certain chemical forces. In absorbing them, the organism transforms them at once into their opposite. This is necessary. If, for example, the food maintained its external character too long after being absorbed, then it would begin to break down as it does in outer nature and would thus introduce destructive and death-bringing processes into the human being. What enters the human being with the foodstuffs, has to be met immediately by inner processes and be transformed into its opposite.

You can pursue the details of processes that I have described for you here through the entire human being. Let us assume, for example, that you stick a foreign object like a splinter into yourself [*see drawing 3, yellow*]. Your

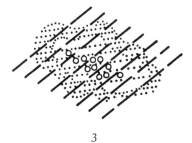

3

body can react to this foreign body in two ways. Suppose you cannot extract the foreign object, that it remains inside you. Then two things can happen. The constructive force active in the flowing blood surrounds the foreign object [*red*]. It gathers around the 'intruder', but in doing so it moves away from its own customary position. This immediately leads to a preponderance of the nerve activity there. Then an exudate-like formation begins to encapsulate the foreign object [*blue*]. Because of this cyst formation, the following takes place in that part of the body. Whereas usually, when there is not a foreign object in that spot, the etheric body penetrates the physical body in a certain way, in this situation the etheric body is unable to penetrate the foreign object; instead, within this area a blister or cyst will form that is filled out only with the etheric [*see drawing, red lines*]. Thus a part of our body contains a foreign object where a small portion of the etheric body is not organized by the physical. In this case it is important to strengthen the astral body in that spot to such an extent that it can be effective in the small portion of the etheric body without the help of the physical body. Through this encapsulation our body has actually made use of the destructive forces, separating out these destructive forces in a small section of the body and then incorporating into it the healing etheric body. This activity will then need to be supported by the astral and the ego through an appropriate treatment.

In such a case we have to say that, in a certain sense, what lies above the physical in the human being has to become strong enough to be active without the physical in this small part of the human organization. This always happens in the healing of some foreign intrusion in the human being, for example when a person gets stuck with a splinter and it becomes encapsulated. In this part of his body man's whole organization is moved up a level as it were. It can also happen that something foreign is formed purely out of the organism. This must be regarded in the same way.

A completely different process could take place, however, if we have a splinter in us. It could be that the nerve activity surrounding the splinter gets stronger and predominates over the blood activity [see drawing 4, yellow]. Then the nerve activity, in which the ego is active (or possibly the ego strengthened by the astral body), stimulates the blood activity. The nerve-sense activity, which penetrates the whole body, stimulates the blood activity and does not permit an exudate to coagulate. Instead it stimulates a secretory process, leading to the formation of

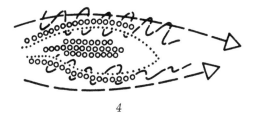

4

pus (white). And because the nerves push through to the outside [*arrows*], the pus is also driven to the periphery by the thrust that goes through the nerve tracts in their breaking down activity. The splinter suppurates out, comes out and the area heals over.

You can see immediately in these processes of encapsulation what occurs specifically when the splinter is too deep in the organism, so that the pushing force of the breaking down, catabolic system, the nerve-sense system, is insufficient to bring it to the outside; then the constructive activity in the blood vessels will be stronger and lead to encapsulation instead.

If the splinter is closer to the surface, then the pushing force of the nerves, the catabolic force, will be stronger. It will excite or stimulate the substance that then becomes an exudate so that it will make use of the catabolic paths that are always present anyway, leading to the outside, and the whole area will suppurate. Therefore we can actually say that we carry in us, in incipient form, in the moment of coming into being, the tendency for our organism to harden towards the inside, in a centripetal direction, and to dissolve again towards the outside in a centrifugal direction. In the normal processes of the human body, however, the tumour-forming force that is directed inwards and the suppurating inflammatory force that is directed towards the periphery are in equilibrium. Generally our inflammatory process is strong enough to counter the tumour-forming, catabolic force. Only when one process is stronger than the other will an actual tumour-formation or an actual inflammation develop.

Now, don't think that all this works out as easily and simply in reality as we necessarily have to present it in schematic description. In reality, these processes are meshed. For example, you know that when the inflammatory forces are strong, we also often have a fever. Basically this is caused by overly strong, excessive anabolic processes in the blood. Indeed, the forces we often develop during a fever would almost be sufficient to supply energy for another person if they could be conducted there.

On the other hand, when the catabolic forces predominate, we have cold symptoms, which are not as easy to diagnose as a fever. Of course, sometimes the two conditions alternate, and so, in practice, we often have to deal with an intermingling of what we really need to keep separate to fully understand the matter.

A question often arises concerning poisons that occur in nature, for example the poison in belladonna, the deadly nightshade: how are actual poisons different from ordinary substances that we find in our environment and use for food?

When we eat food, something is introduced into the organism that is formed in outer nature similarly to the way in which our invisible human being is formed. We take into us something that proceeds from a spiritual activity [*see drawing 5, yellow*], enters an astral activity [*red*], then an etheric activity (blue), and finally a physical activity [*white*]. In nature such an activity is directed from

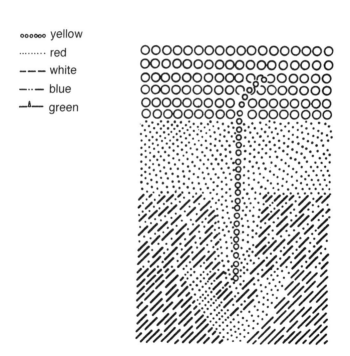

above downwards; it acts upon the earth from the periphery, as it were. This activity is related to our inner ego activity, which is a purely spiritual activity. If what I have drawn schematically as yellow flows down but transforms itself via the astral, then further via the etheric, then down into the physical, the plant as a rule takes up such an activity. The plant grows towards this activity from below upwards and takes up this etheric activity, which, however, already inherently contains from above the astral and ego activity, i.e., soul and spiritual activity.

It is also possible for something else to take place, as it does with a poison. Poisonous substances have the peculiarity that they do not make use of the etheric as do the normal green substances in the plant; instead they turn directly to the astral, so that the astral, which I have drawn in red here, enters into this substance [*see colour drawing 5, lower red in white*]. With belladonna, the fruit becomes extraordinarily greedy and because of this greed is not satisfied by taking up just the etheric; instead the fruit takes up the astral directly, before this astral has taken up the etheric life forces in streaming downwards. You could say that in such cases the astral is continually dripping from the world-periphery directly down to the earth instead of first entering the etheric. And such drops of the astral being, which have not gone through the ether atmosphere of the earth in the right way, can, for example, be found in the poison of the deadly nightshade. We also have this cosmic, astral element dripping down into the plant in the poison of the thorn apple (*Datura*) in the *Hyoscyamus*, the poison of the henbane, etc.

What therefore lives in this plant substance, for example in the deadly nightshade, is related to the activity that enters the human nerves and circulation of oxygen directly from the ego or the astral body. Thus by absorbing the poison of the deadly nightshade, we get a significant strengthening of the catabolic processes in us, those processes that otherwise enter the physical body directly from the ego. The human ego is not generally strong enough to tolerate such a strengthening of catabolic processes. If the opposing activity is too great, however, the activity that proceeds from below upwards in the blood vessels can be countered with such catabolic processes derived from nature. Atropine, the poison of the deadly nightshade, can thus be used in small doses to counteract overly strong growth processes in the human being. The moment there is too much of this poison, however, we cannot speak any longer of equilibrium. Then, to begin with, growth processes are pushed back, and the human being is numbed by a spiritual activity that he is not yet able to tolerate with his ego. He will be able to tolerate such a spiritual activity perhaps only in future conditions, in the Venus and Vulcan stages of evolution.[2] This is why the peculiar symptoms of poisoning occur. First the point of origin of the activity effective in the blood is undermined; then the gastric manifestations arise that appear after the ingestion of deadly nightshade poison; then the forces working from below upwards are strongly prevented from doing so in the right way; and finally, complete loss of consciousness occurs, the destruction of the human being through rampant catabolic processes [...]

Schematic summary:

INVISIBLE MAN FORCES	DIRECT EGO FORCES
Metabolic-limb system	Sense and nervous system
Anabolic (upbuilding)	Catabolic (breaking down)
Works upwards	Works downwards
Unconscious	Conscious
Relaxation	Tension
Fever (hot)	Degenerative, hardening illness (cold)
Exercise, movement	Rest
Centrifugal	Centripetal

8. Cancer and Mistletoe, and Aspects of Psychiatry

In the previous lecture we touched on the nature of cancer from the perspective of the supersensible bodies. There cancer was seen to be linked to dominance of the nerve-sense system. We saw how cancer patients often show an acquiescent response to external demands. In the following passages – also key ones for understanding anthroposophical medicine – Steiner presents a dynamic picture of cancer in terms of the supersensible bodies, and explains why the mistletoe plant could act as an effective remedy. He also describes aspects of mental illness and claims these are rooted not primarily in the brain but in other organs of the body.

In cancer, as Steiner describes it, the etheric body is no longer fully under the influence of the astral and ego, but starts behaving autonomously like a piece of tissue culture separated from the body and growing in a separate nutrient fluid.[1] We could say that cancer is a tissue growing with a foreign etheric force separated from the patient's overall etheric forces; in other words it is no longer under the organism's dominion. There is a lack of apoptosis, or physiological control of growth.

In the last excerpt in this chapter Steiner likens tumour growths to misplaced sensory organs, just as he regards cancer in general as related to a predominance of the nerve-sense system. He also speaks of ways in which we can view medicinal herbs, through an intuitive type of perception that perceives characteristics in them similar to human soul forces. Steiner describes mistletoe as 'aristocratic, Bohemian and contrary'. One could also add that it has a certain maverick quality, doing its own thing – the opposite of many cancer patients who tend to conform and do not quite know what they want to get out of life (Le Shan). In this way Steiner lifts the nature of cancer out of a purely physical view, at the same time raising mistletoe characteristics to the realm of soul pictures – where it proves to be the polar opposite of cancer and therefore exactly what the cancer patient needs for healing.

Although few of us, if any, have Steiner's highly developed perceptive capacities, we can at least make a start in this direction. We can also subject his findings to scientific analysis. Very extensive research has been done on mistletoe (Viscum album), and it has been shown to contain chemical constituents that are cancerostatic and also strengthen the immune system against cancer. A large scientific trial on Viscum album was published in 2001, showing a general increase of survival rate amongst cancer patients of 40% compared to control patients.[2]

Especially with regard to three sets of facts that we must now begin to discuss, the more materialistic trend in medicine may possibly begin to turn towards our spiritual-scientifically oriented school of thought. This will most probably be the case with our observations of everything involved in tumour formation and possible cures for cancer, a truly rational view of so-called mental illnesses, and our knowledge of the therapeutic use of external remedies – liniments, ointments, and the like. We can scarcely hope that conventional physical examinations unguided by spiritual scientific insights will suffice to approach subjects such as the development of growths that culminate in carcinomas. Connections are omnipresent in the natural world, and today's psychiatry is in such a sorry state because there is no human, conscious connection between it and conventional pathology and therapy – two fields that are perhaps the most receptive to spiritual-scientific viewpoints. It will be especially necessary to consider everything spiritual science can say about these topics. Today all that is needed is to consider my writings; you will find that they have already said quite a lot in this regard. We need to take into account all aspects of the etheric body's intervention in the human organism.

It should not be said that clairvoyance is absolutely necessary in order to be able to talk about the etheric body's activity in the human organism, because a great many processes that simply oppose the etheric body's activities demonstrate that it is not active, or at least not properly active, in a specific way. To come to valid ideas on this subject, we will need to look at inflammations and their consequences as well as at tumour development as initiating the destruction of the human organism, so to speak. In the case of tumour development, very justifiable attempts are now being made to avoid surgery. Because of social circumstances that will need to be changed – not outer conditions, but social circumstances in which medicine plays a part, namely, issues of public health care—this very justified ideal cannot always be implemented. The important point here is to create a substitute for what the surgeon's knife does or does not accomplish—and it certainly is effective in some respects but fails to accomplish anything in others. There are undoubtedly many people who advocate surgery today simply because they have no way of knowing about anything else but who will immediately take the opposite approach as soon as information becomes available.

You do not need me to describe the character of inflammatory processes in their various specific forms organ by organ. I am sure this is well known, but what is not so well known is the overriding process common to all inflammatory processes. This common process can best be characterized by saying that in every true inflammation, whether very small or very large, and in everything that can lead from inflammation to ulceration, spiritual scientific investigation will reveal that the human etheric body as a whole is still functioning. This means that we can count on being able to do something to normalize and redistribute the etheric body's effect, which has become sluggish in a single direction, so that the person's entire etheric body will then work in a healthy way. In inflammations, the etheric body's activity is guided only in specific directions, whereas the activity of a healthy etheric body extends into the organism in all the appropriate directions. In essence, we can say that if the etheric body as a whole is still healthy but has become sluggish with regard to a particular organ system, we will be able to discover agents, which we will discuss later, that are capable of stimulating it to develop its universal activity, if I may call it that, in this specific direction.

It is different in tumour formations of any sort. In this case, certain processes in the physical body function directly as enemies of the etheric body's activity. These processes in the physical body simply rebel against the etheric body's activity. As a consequence, the etheric body is no longer effective in these areas of the physical body. The etheric body, however, has a great capacity for regeneration, and spiritual-scientific observation always shows that if we can remove the obstruction and overcome the enemy that counteracts the etheric body's activity in a certain area, we will indeed be able to deal with the problem. With tumours, then, it is a matter of using natural processes to stimulate the removal of the physical processes opposing the etheric body so that it can once again work in a location its effects formerly could not reach.

This will become very important in the treatment of carcinomas. If carcinomas are observed objectively it is quite evident that, in spite of their many different forms, they all constitute a revolt on the part of certain physical forces against the forces of the etheric body. The keratinization that typically appears in internal carcinomas and is less prominent in carcinomas located nearer the surface—although the tendency persists—shows us that a physical formative process has overcome the etheric formative process that should be present at that particular spot.

A careful study of these two phenomena — inflammation and ulceration on the one hand and tumour formation on the other — eventually makes it obvious that they are true polar opposites. Having said that this is obvious, let me also ask you to recall your experience of carcinomas located close to the surface. What happens in such cases can frequently be confused with pseudo-abscesses, at least in certain respects. Above all, therefore, it will be important to study this polarity more precisely.

Medical nomenclature that is at least medieval, if not exactly ancient, is often very disturbing in such instances. I am not referring to the historical medieval period but to the Middle Ages of nomenclature that lie in the quite recent past. It is not totally correct to describe tumours as 'neoplasms'. There is nothing new about them except in the very trivial sense of not having been there before; they are not new in the sense of growing out of the skin-enclosed organism of their own accord. They come about because the physical body counters the etheric body so strongly that the outer body aligns itself with aspects of outer nature that are inimical to the human being. Tumour development offers easy access to all sorts of outer influences.

Here again it is important to study the image that contrasts with all these processes. Let me point you first in the direction of studying the development of *Viscum* (mistletoe) in outer nature. Although we do initially need to pay attention to how *Viscum* species develop on other plants, this is not the most important consideration. The parasitic nature of mistletoe is certainly the most important consideration for botany, but as far as our study of the connection between outer, non-human nature and the human being is concerned, a much more important consideration is that mistletoe, because it grows on other plants, on trees, is forced to carry out its vegetative growth in a different annual rhythm. For example, it has already finished flowering before the trees it grows on have begun putting out leaves in spring. It is a winter plant and rather aristocratic in its behaviour. It uses the foliage of its host trees to protect it from the intense light of summer and does not expose itself to the most intense rays of the sun. (In line with the processes we described the day before yesterday, we must always see the sun simply as a representative of the effects of light, but this would need to be studied in the context of physics and does not belong in this discussion. We cannot completely avoid what has crept into our language as a result of somewhat inaccurate observations of nature.)

Mistletoe's whole way of growing and thriving by attaching itself to other plants is especially important because it allows this plant to acquire very specific forces that can be described more or less as follows. Thanks to the forces it acquires, it rejects the intentions of organisational forces that develop in a straight line and demands their opposite. Here, too, the situation will become clear only when we understand it in the following way. Here is a schematic representation [*see blackboard sketch*] of a spot in the human body that uses its own forces to revolt against all the etheric forces working into it. The etheric forces are dammed up and brought to a standstill, and as a result something that looks like a new growth comes about. Mistletoe is a remedy that counteracts the etheric pocket that has formed here. It pulls the etheric forces back into this spot where they did not want to go.

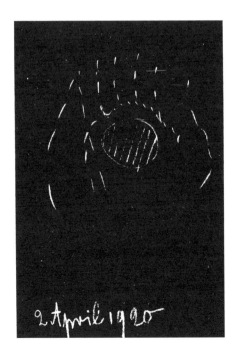

2 April 1920

You will be able to convince yourselves of this situation through an experiment that can be performed only by taking advantage of a coincidental opportunity. You will be able to study mistletoe's tendency to oppose straight-line organization if you have an opportunity to observe its effect on the expulsion of the placenta. Mistletoe causes the placenta to be retained in the human organism; that is, in its own way it does the opposite of what straight-line organization wants. The ability to cause retention of the placenta — that is, to bring the usual organizational process to a standstill — is one of the most important characteristics of mistletoe's effective processes. Of course, in the case of more subtle activities in the human organism that have the same basis as placental retention, this effect is much less readily apparent, but the same force that is strongly active when mistletoe counteracts the straight-line organizational tendency also confronts us in any other images we get of mistletoe's effect. Having noticed that mistletoe counters the etheric body's failure to take hold of the physical body to the right extent, if we then induce a specific mistletoe effect, the etheric body may take hold of the physical body too strongly, resulting in convulsions. In other cases, the effects of mistletoe can cause the peculiar sensation of being in constant danger of falling over. These consequences are also related to the fact that mistletoe essentially promotes nocturnal emissions, among other things. ·

You can see in every instance — even in connection with the development of epilepsy, for example — that mistletoe has the capacity of opposing the human organism. This ability has less to do with the fact that it is a parasite, however, than with the fact that it allows nature to 'give it an extra helping of sausage'[3] — to use an expression that at least the Viennese among you will understand. It is granted a special favour, an exception to the rule, in that it refuses to thrive in the usual season, to flower in the spring and then bear fruit. Instead, it does these things in a different season, during the winter. By doing so, it retains forces that then counteract the normal course of events. If it is not too offensive, we may say that if we look at how nature behaves in the development of mistletoe, nature seems to have gone crazy. It does everything at the wrong time when it comes to mistletoe. This behaviour, however, is exactly what we will put to use when the human organism goes physically crazy, which is what happens in the development of carcinomas. The point is to develop an understanding of such relationships.

There can be no doubt that mistletoe is the substance that, if potentized,[4] will allow us to replace the surgeon's knife in treating tumours. It is only a question of handling mistletoe fruit in the right way — but in connection with other forces in mistletoe itself, of course — so as to turn it into a remedy.

Mistletoe's craziness is also evident in the fact that its continued existence and reproduction are always dependent on being moved from place to place by birds. Mistletoe would surely die out if birds did not repeatedly carry its means of reproduction from one tree to another.

Curiously enough, its reproductive structures also choose to pass through the birds themselves, in that they are first taken into the birds' bodies and later evacuated so that they can sprout on another tree. All these findings, if observed objectively, lead to insight into mistletoe's entire process of development. The gluey substance in mistletoe, in particular, needs to be brought into the right connection with a triturating (or bulking) agent so as to gradually produce a very high potency of this substance.

Next, this substance needs to be specially adapted to different organs—I will go into detail later—in part by considering the origin of the mistletoe, specifically what kind of a tree it grew on. But it will also be important to produce remedies that are based on the interaction of this gluey substance with specific metallic substances, which can even be derived from the metal content of other plants. For example, the interaction that comes about by combining and potentizing mistletoe from apple trees with silver salts will result in a remedy that can be highly effective against all abdominal cancers.

You must understand that I need to speak cautiously about these subjects, because although the basic thrust of what I am saying is absolutely correct and well founded in spiritual-scientific research, actual therapeutic measures depend totally on how mistletoe's constituents are processed, and the knowledge needed to produce such remedies is scarcely available yet. At this point, of course, spiritual science would be able to work favourably only when it could actually constantly collaborate with the clinical process that is the basis of so much of what other physicians do. This is what makes the relationship between spiritual science and medicine so difficult. These two approaches—the opportunity for clinical observation and spiritual-scientific research—are forced to remain separated because of modern social conventions. It will become evident that we will get nowhere unless these two paths are brought together. The important point will be to gather empirical evidence, because the only way you will be able to impress the outer world is if you can at least supply verification in the form of outer clinical reports and so on. The need for these proofs is more an outer than an inner one.

If we simply proceed methodically, we will be able to prove that the effect of mistletoe really is based on what I have just explained. According to what I said here a few days ago, tree trunks are more like outgrowths of soil substance, little hills in which the vegetative aspect is still present and which support the growth of everything else that belongs to the tree. When mistletoe also grows there, its roots grow towards the ground as it makes itself at home up there on the tree. Thus it is to be expected that if we conduct experiments with plants that have the same crazy aristocratic attitude as mistletoe but lack its Bohemian parasitic quality, we will see similar characteristics—and this is indeed the case. If we begin to investigate winter plants with regard to their tendency to counteract normal tendencies of the human organism, and specifically normal tendencies to develop illnesses, we can expect that plants that find it appropriate to put forth flowers in winter will all have similar effects. For example, if we simply extend our experiments to include *Helleborus niger,* the common Christmas rose, we will find that it induces similar effects. We must take into account, however, the contrast between male and female that I have at least begun to characterize. With *Helleborus niger,* we can hardly expect to achieve clearly visible results in women, but results will be perceptible in cases of tumour development in men if we use a similar processing method but produce a higher potency than the one I indicated in the case of *Viscum.*

If we work in this way, we must consider relationships of this sort—whether a plant thrives in winter or summer, whether it derives its effect from behaving like mistletoe or whether it is more inclined towards the earth. Mistletoe does not like to be close to the earth, but black hellebore, or Christmas rose, does and is therefore more closely related to the male system of forces, which in turn is more closely related to earthly factors, as I explained a few days ago. The female system of forces is instead more closely connected to supra-earthly factors. These differences absolutely must be taken into account. It will prove especially important to acquire a certain insight into the processes of nature. This is why, in the attempt to illustrate the forces in the outer world, I turned to concepts of character such as 'Bohemian', 'aristocratic', and 'crazy' (which can serve us very well and are not at all inadequate with respect to what we are considering) to show what these forces are like.

Having acquired such concepts, we will then encounter the characteristic difference between a remedy's external and internal effects. But before we take this difference into account, we must also look at ideas that can introduce it in the right way. For example, there is one thing that will absolutely have to be studied with regard to certain illnesses that are now appearing. In the case of these new types of illness, which I pointed out yesterday, we will have to study what happens, for example, when we expose *Carbo vegetabilis* to marsh gas for some time simply by leaving it lying in the gas; we proceed with trituration only after the carbon is sufficiently impregnated with gas. The result will be externally effective in some way, in the form of ointments and the like, especially if the trituration is performed in conjunction with substances that can enhance the effect further. It is simply a question of discovering the right technique. If triturated with talc, for example, according to certain technical methods that we will certainly be able to ascertain, the resulting remedy will be very effective if used externally in the form of ointments and suchlike.

The important thing for us now, however, is to understand such a process. We will not understand it if we do not first sharpen our vision by learning healthy thinking with regard to psychiatry. Please believe me that spiritual scientists are actually angered, if I may express myself drastically, by the use of the German word *Geisteskrankheit* ('spirit illness') for psychiatric illness. It is ridiculous to use this term because the spirit is always healthy and incapable of falling ill. What happens is that the spirit's ability to express itself is disturbed by the physical organism. There is never any real illness in the life of the spirit or soul. Symptoms appear, but that is all.

Now, however, we must sharpen our vision for specific individual symptoms. Perhaps you will see the first indications and then the further development of something like religious mania. (As you know, these terms are not all precise because the nomenclature in this field is extremely confused. Nevertheless, we do need to use these words.) All this, of course, is merely symptomatic. But assuming that something like this develops, the important point will be to gain a picture of its entire process of development. Once we have acquired this picture, however, and encounter an individual with this symptomatology, we will have to look carefully at any abnormalities in the process of lung formation—not in the respiratory process, but in the lungs' formative process, in pulmonary metabolism. You see, the term brain disease is also not totally correct. If the term *Geisteskrankheit* is completely false, then 'brain disease' is actually half false, because any degeneration in the brain is always secondary. The primary factor in all psychiatric illnesses never lies in the upper part of the body, but always in the lower part, in the organs belonging to the four systems of the liver, kidneys, heart and lungs. In the case of someone who is losing interest in outer life and beginning to brood and act out delusions, the most important concern is always to get an idea of the constitution of this person's pulmonary process. This is extremely important.

Similarly, if we observe someone in whom obstinacy, pigheadedness, and self-righteousness appear, indicating a certain immobility or rigidity in thinking, this should lead us to investigate the status of liver function in the person in question. In such people, it is always the inner organic chemistry that is not functioning properly. Even what we have become accustomed to calling 'softening of the brain' in common parlance is entirely secondary. The primary factor in psychiatric disorders, even if it is sometimes more difficult to observe, always lies in the lower organ systems. This accounts for the often dishearteningly low rate of success of psychotherapy. In fact, psychotherapy can accomplish more in the case of organic diseases than it can in so-called psychiatric disorders. We will have to get used to treating psychiatric disorders with medical remedies.[5] This is crucial, and it is the second of two areas in which outer trends in medicine will have to find a way to approach spiritual science.

In this area, well-trained psychologists will always prove to be the best observers. An extraordinary amount lies hidden in our psychological life, with all its great variety and its frequently merely suggestive effects. We will gradually have to achieve a real capacity for observation in this field. It is not true that human beings are simple or simply constituted in terms of their abilities, by which I also mean the capacities of the bodily state of organization, which is the tool of a person's spiritual organization. Let me give an example. Strange as it may sound, it is absolutely possible for someone we are obliged to describe as an idiot, as a feebleminded person, to have abilities that allow him or her to come up with comments that are witty and brilliant. This is truly possible, because feeblemindedness can make a person very open to suggestion, very receptive to reflecting the mysterious influences of his or her surroundings. There are very interesting observations to be made in the field of pathology and cultural history. We must not name names in reporting the results of such observations, which would detract from their credibility. It is not right to name names, but it is an idiosyncrasy of the field of journalism in particular that people with feeble minds can become good journalists because their slow wit puts them in a position to reflect the opinion of the times rather than giving their own obstinate views. For example, dull-witted journalists reflect the opinion of the times to such an extent that their accounts are much more interesting than those of self-possessed, strong-minded journalists. We learn much more about what humanity as a whole is thinking from weak-minded journalists than from strong-minded ones, who are always intent on developing opinions of their own.

This is an extreme case, but it occurs over and over again. It is the ultimate disguise of the actual state of affairs. We fail to notice the presence of feeblemindedness because its initial manifestation can be quite brilliant. In everyday life such a circumstance doesn't make much difference. Ultimately, no harm is done if our newspapers are written by the feebleminded, as long as they present only good things. In extreme cases, however, where the limit is reached and this tendency develops into a form of illness, we need to acquire a very unbiased eye for observing the soul conditions of people who then fall into the domain of psychiatry. Since we will not always be able to judge by the disguises their soul activity has assumed, we will have to make our assessments on the basis of deeper-lying symptoms.

We must always realize that it is easiest of all to succumb to error when we are observing psychological states, because the most important question is not whether the person expresses intelligent thoughts, for example, but whether he or she tends to repeat these intelligent thoughts more often than the context necessitates. *How* an individual expresses his or her thoughts is the important thing. Whether a person repeats thoughts very frequently or utters them without supplying transitions is more important than whether the thoughts themselves are intelligent or stupid. A completely healthy person can still be stupid—merely physiologically stupid, not pathologically stupid. It is also possible for someone to express a clever thought and still be predisposed to psychiatric illness and even succumb to it. We can see this most readily if the person in question suffers from omission of thoughts or frequent repetition of thoughts The person who suffers from frequent repetitions always has a potential for illness that is related to a formative lung process that is not in order, while the one who suffers from omission of thoughts always has an inherent predisposition to a liver process that is not functioning properly. Other symptoms fall in between these two extremes.

These questions, too, can be studied in real life, for example, in cases where a substance is used for pleasure rather than as a medicine, at least in the ordinary sense. We can see that coffee has a very clear and pronounced effect on the entire symptomatic process of our psychological life (I have often mentioned this before, in certain circles). We should not value such effects, although they are indeed present, because reliance on them simply makes the soul sluggish. It is possible to compensate for deficient logic by consuming coffee, that is, coffee consumption predisposes the organism to release more forces for purposes of logic than is the case when a person does not drink coffee. Thus, drinking a lot of coffee is one of the habits of modern journalists, which means they have to chew on their pens less in order to connect one thought to another.

This is one aspect of the question. In contrast, tea consumption prevents us from always linking one thought to the next in a pedantic, professorial fashion, which, if taken to extremes, is not at all witty but bores people because we are constantly subjecting them to the precision of our own logical processes. Certain professions are now in decline, but they might have made good use of an external means of becoming as witty as possible without inwardly being so. Members of these professions should have been advised to drink tea. Just as coffee is a good drink for journalists, tea is an extremely effective drink for diplomats, who have great need of the ability to habitually toss off disjointed thoughts that allow one to appear witty.

Such things are important to know, because if we can acknowledge them properly and have the necessary moral attitude of soul, we know as a matter of course that these abilities must be promoted in some other, non-dietary way. Such connections are extraordinarily important as a means of educating ourselves about certain natural relationships. Similarly, in a cultural context, it is important to look, for example, at the very low sugar consumption that was once typical in Russia, in contrast to the very high consumption typical in the Western or English-speaking world. We will discover that where psychological development has not overtaken such manifestations, people present a very clear imprint of what they ingest. Russians express a certain selfless devotion to the outer world and have less ego awareness, which they substitute for on a level that is theoretical at best. This is related to low sugar consumption. In contrast, the British possess a strong, organically based sense of self that is related to high sugar consumption. Here, however, it is less important to look at actual consumption levels than at people's sugar cravings, because the level of consumption always develops as the result of a craving, out of the longing to enjoy something. That is why it is especially important to take a look at such cravings.

Looking to the organ systems of the lower human body,

as the origin of so-called psychiatric disorders, points us in the direction of interactions within the human being that should not be disregarded from the joint perspective of pathology and therapy. These interactions between what I have described in simple terms as the upper and lower areas of the human being must always be taken into account with regard to both pathology and therapy. If we neglect to do so, we will never achieve a proper view of the effect of outer influences through which we want to work on a patient. It makes a big difference whether we apply the effects of warmth or water to a patient's feet or head. But we cannot bring reason to bear on these questions without first becoming aware of the great differences in the functioning of the upper and lower parts of the human being. This is why we will now discuss outer effects on the human being, to the extent that our particular subject permits.

This next excerpt from another lecture describes how in cancer etheric forces of growth are not properly kept in check by the other supersensible aspects of the human being. Steiner also describes what happens when the astral body becomes too dominant.

Let me give two brief examples to elucidate the spiritual and practical ramifications of what I have already presented. Let us assume that spiritual diagnosis—if I may call it that—shows that a person's etheric body predominates in a particular part of the body and that its activity is too strong. Spiritual vision confronts us with the fact that the etheric body is working too hard in one organ. Neither the astral body's catabolic processes nor re-enlivening by the ego controls the etheric body's over-whelming process in this particular organ. We see an astral organization that is too weak and possibly also an inadequately directed ego. Consequently, the etheric body predominates in this particular organ. The processes of growth and nutrition are so forceful that the human organism is inadequately controlled by the astral body and the 'I'.

At this location in the dominant etheric body, the human body seems too strongly exposed to centrifugal forces working out into the cosmos. These forces, which are active in the etheric body, are out of balance with the centripetal forces of the physical body, and the astral body cannot control the resulting developments. In this case, we are faced with both a predominance of the activity of silica and the ego's inability to control it. Such phenomena, which are always present when tumours develop, enable us to truly understand cancer.

As you may know, cancer research has resulted in some very promising treatments, and its successes are as great as any that are possible on a physical level. But we cannot understand cancers as long as we do not know that they involve a predominance of the etheric body that is not forced back or broken down by appropriate activity of the astral body or ego. Then the question arises of what we must do to strengthen the astral body and ego in this particular organ so that the predominance of the etheric body can be adequately broken down. This is an initial abstract formulation of the question that set us on the path to the cancer therapy that I will discuss tomorrow. In this instance, understanding the etheric body opens a way for us to learn to comprehend one of the worst human illnesses and to combat it by discerning the spiritual effects of remedies. This is an example of a case where we must look at the etheric body in order to understand the illness completely.[6]

Next, let's assume that the astral body predominates throughout most of the body. We see a general stiffening of the astral body, so to speak. It becomes excessively forceful, and it takes itself more seriously than it deserves in the context of the entire organism. What are the consequences when the astral body cannot be controlled by the 'I', when its degenerative, catabolic processes are not neutralized and balanced by appropriate re-enlivening? The resulting symptoms have to do primarily with ego weakness, because when the astral body is too strong the 'I' is proportionally too weak. Symptoms that stem from weakness of the ego are also always related to an excessively strong astral body.

Chief among these symptoms is abnormal cardiac activity, so we must look for a syndrome that includes it. Another consequence of 'I'-activity that is too weak in proportion to the astral body is increased glandular activity. The functions of glands close to the body's surface begin to predominate, because they are inadequately controlled by the ego. For example, goitre may develop, causing swelling of the glands in the throat. In addition, because the 'I'-organization is unable to work strongly enough (especially in the sensory organs), the stiffening of the astral body forces the activity of silica outwards — which ought in fact to work back from within. Consequently, we find that the patient's eyes protrude. The astral body forces the eyes outwards, and the function of the ego is to counteract this protruding tendency. Our eyes are held in place by the stable but delicate balance between the ego and the astral body. When a patient's eyes protrude as if attempting to escape from the body, we know that the ego is too weak to keep them in their proper place. Other symptoms, such as general restlessness, sensitivity and nervousness, also indicate a preponderance of the astral body's activity, because the 'I' cannot adequately repress the organic processes the astral body induces. When the ego is too weak and the patient is pushed around by the astral body, which should be subordinate to the 'I', the symptoms include insomnia, protruding eves and abnormal glandular activity — in short, the symptoms of Graves' disease [*hyperthyroidism, or exophthalmic goitre*]. Having realized that Graves' disease is induced by a disturbance in the balance between ego and astral body, we can attempt to develop an appropriate treatment. As you see, both the pathological condition and its treatment can be studied with great precision with the help of spiritual insight into the human being.

I have now completed my introduction and hope to

move on tomorrow, using the two examples I have just given to demonstrate how spiritual diagnostics leads to spiritual treatments. I will use the two characteristic syndromes of cancer and Graves' disease to show how a truly exact spiritual foundation for both pathology and treatment enriches and complements conventional medical therapies. Treatments for these two syndromes will serve as the basis for providing a more complete picture of therapy in general. Now let us ask what we must do in the case of cancer. Yesterday, we discussed how the etheric body develops too much strength in a particular organ. The centrifugal forces, the forces that want to move out into the cosmos, become excessively strong, and the astral body and ego are unable to counteract them sufficiently. At this point, spiritual insight tells us that either we must attempt to strengthen the astral body by turning to the plant kingdom or we must suppress the effects of the etheric body by turning to the animal kingdom.[7] The initial results of our spiritual research prompted us to attempt to cure cancer by strengthening the astral body. When we look for any remedy that affects the astral body, we must look in the plant kingdom, and, in fact, our cancer remedy was discovered there.

We have been accused of introducing all kinds of amateurish ideas into our efforts, because our first step towards finding a cure for cancer involved specially processed mistletoe, a parasitic plant that is otherwise used medicinally only in the treatment of epilepsy and similar disorders. Mistletoe, however, is a very special plant.

Look at trees with strange tumour-like outgrowths emerging from their bark. The normally vertical growth tendency is diverted at a right angle and assumes a horizontal direction, as if a second trunk were beginning to grow outwards. In effect, the tree is parasitizing itself. By studying this phenomenon more closely, you find that the physical body of the tree above the burl is always negatively affected. Because the physical substance that gets through is not enough to allow the physical body to accommodate the etheric body's forces of growth, the tree's physical body is retarded. The etheric body, whose centrifugal forces normally attempt to fling physical matter out into the cosmos, is left to its own devices in the portion of the tree above the outgrowth [*see drawing*]. Too

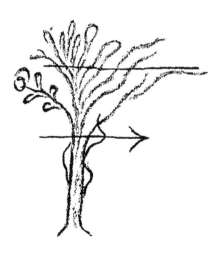

little physical substance, or at least substance with too little physical energy, gets through. As a result, the etheric body turns back towards the stronger, lower part of the tree. In essence, therefore, the etheric body becomes too strong.

Now imagine instead that a parasitic mistletoe plant establishes itself at the same location. The same phenomenon occurs, but it is caused by a second plant with its own etheric body rather than by the tree's etheric body. As a result, the mistletoe develops a very specific relationship to the tree. The tree, which is grounded in the soil, assimilates forces from the soil. The mistletoe, which is attached to the tree, assimilates what the tree supplies; that is, it uses the tree as its soil. Mistletoe artificially brings about the same preponderance of the tree's etheric body that occurs naturally in outgrowths. What mistletoe takes from the tree is available only when the tree has a deficiency of physical substance and an excess of the etheric aspect. The etheric excess moves from the tree into

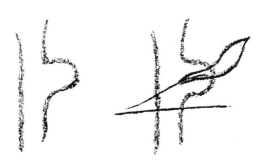

the mistletoe. Inner vision reveals that when we process mistletoe in a way that allows this etheric excess to be transferred to a human being — via injection, under certain circumstances — mistletoe, as a foreign substance, takes over for the cancer's rampant etheric substance and strengthens the effect of the patient's astral body by suppressing the physical cancer, causing the tumour to disintegrate. When we administer mistletoe substances, we use them as a vehicle for the tree's etheric substance. The actual remedy is etheric tree substance, which strengthens the human astral body.

   This method requires insight into how a plant's etheric body influences the human astral body — specifically, how the spiritual aspect of the tree that is drawn out by the parasitic plant affects the astral aspect in the human being. The example of mistletoe supplies concrete confirmation of what I said yesterday, namely, that when we use medicinal substances we are using not only what chemistry knows about them but also the spirit that is present in them.

The next excerpt draws parallels between tumour formation and a 'sense organ in the wrong place'. Another way to see this is that a kind of consciousness penetrates areas where it does not belong.

Please note that everything I am saying here in a physiological sense is of importance for pathology and therapy. When we observe this intricate organism of man we find, of course, that one system of organs is continually pouring out its influences into another system of organs. If we now observe the whole dynamic action expressed in one of the sense organs, in the ear for example, we find the following: ego organization and astral, etheric and physical organization are all working together in a specific way. The metabolism permeates the nerves and senses; rhythm is introduced into this by the processes of breathing, in so far as these work into the ear, and by the blood circulation. All that I have tried to describe to you in diverse ways, in terms of threefold and fourfold levels of the human organism, finds expression in definite relationships in every single organ. In the long run, all things in man are in constant metamorphosis and dynamic flux.

For instance, why do we call normal what normally occurs in the region of the ear? Because it appears precisely as it does in order that the human being as a whole, even as he lives and moves on earth, may come into existence. We have no other reason to call it normal. But consider now the special circumstances, the special formative forces that work here in the ear by virtue of the ear's position, by virtue of the fact that the ear is at the periphery of the organism. Suppose that these circumstances are working in such a way that a similar relationship arises by metamorphosis, at some other place in the interior of the body. Instead of the relationship which is proper to that place in the body there arises a relationship among the various members of the organism similar to what is normal in the region of the ear. Then there will grow at this place in the body something that really tends to become an ear—forgive this very sketchy way of putting it. I cannot express what I want to say in any other way, as I am obliged to describe things in the briefest outline. For instance, this something may grow in the region of the pylorus instead of what should arise there. In a pathological metamorphosis of this kind, we have to see the origins of tumours and similar formations. *All tumour formations and carcinomas are really misplaced attempts to form a sense organ.*

If, then, you bear in mind that the origin of a malignant growth is a misplaced attempt at the formation of a sense organ, you will find what part is played in the child's constitution, even in embryonic development, by the organisms of warmth and air, in order that sense organs may come into being. These organs can indeed only come into being through the organisms of warmth and air, by virtue of the resistance of the solid and fluid organisms, which results in a formation composed of both factors. This means that we must observe the relationship existing between the physical organism (as far as this expresses itself in the metabolism, for example) and the formative, structuring organism (in so far as this expresses itself in the system of nerves and senses). We must, so to speak, perceive how the metabolic system radiates out the forces which bear the substance along with them, and how the substance is shaped and moulded in the organs by the forces brought to meet it by the system of nerves and senses.

Bearing this in mind, we shall learn to understand what

a tumour formation really is. On the one side there is a false relationship between the physical-etheric organism in so far as it expresses itself in the radiating metabolic processes on the one hand, and between the ego organization and astral organism on the other (in so far as the ego and astral organizations express themselves in the warmth and airy organizations respectively). Ultimately, therefore, we have above all to deal with the relation between the metabolism and the warmth organization in man, and in the case of an internal tumour—although it is also possible with a peripheral tumour—the best treatment is to envelop it in warmth. (I shall speak of these things tomorrow when we come to consider therapy). The point is to succeed in enveloping the tumour with warmth. This brings about a radical change in the whole organization. If we succeed in surrounding the tumour with warmth, then, speaking crudely, we shall also succeed in dissolving it. This can actually be achieved by the proper use of certain remedies which are injected into the organism. We may be sure that in every case a preparation of *Viscum*, applied in the way we advise around the abnormal organ—for instance around the tumour growth—will generate a mantle of warmth, only we must first have ascertained its specific effect upon this or that system of organs.

We cannot, of course, apply exactly the same preparation to carcinoma of the breast as to carcinoma of the uterus or of the pylorus. Further, we can be sure that no result will be achieved if we do not succeed in producing the right reaction, namely, a state of feverishness. The injection must be followed by a certain rise in the patient's temperature. You can immediately expect failure if no condition of feverishness is produced.

I wanted to tell you this as a principle in order that you can understand that these things depend on a rationale, but the rationale is merely a regulating principle. You will find that the statements based on this principle can be verified as all such facts are verified by the methods of modern science and medicine. There is no question of asking you to simply accept these things before they have been tested, but it is really true that anyone who studies them carefully can make remarkable discoveries.

Although this brief exposition may be somewhat confusing initially, everything will become clear if you study the subject deeply.

9. Case History Questions: Diagnosis and Therapy

In the following lecture Steiner tells us about certain signs and symptoms and what they reveal about the nature of the super-sensible bodies. He highlights principles that can be employed while taking down a case history and making a diagnosis, though his descriptions of course cover only a fraction of possible symptoms. All signs and symptoms, if we can read them aright, reveal something of the nature of the supersensible bodies.

In this lecture there is also a description of the polar effect of minerals and of the inverse relationship between the human being and the plant world. Steiner describes how this relation-ship helps us to understand how various parts of the plant can work therapeutically.

The following criteria that Steiner refers to are all ones that a practising doctor can draw on to create an overall picture and diagnosis: age, growth and body build, dream life, movement/ inertia, short/long sight, teeth, cravings and aversions – for sugar or salt for instance – vertigo, and disturbances in elim-ination, such as perspiration and urine/bowel movements. All such symptoms can be compiled to form an overall picture of a patient, so that we start to see where the proper actions of the supersensible bodies are obstructed or excessively strong. This unity, which the doctor can create as a picture of the patient, forms the subsequent basis for therapy and natural remedies whose 'pictures' or indications are the opposite of the remedy's therapeutic effect. For instance, the picture of phosphorus is a rich dream life and artistic temperament, but its effect is to help upper supersensible bodies unite more strongly with the lower ones, as Steiner relates later in the lecture.

In the course of these lectures, as we draw ever closer to that special field where pathology penetrates into therapy, bridging the gap between the two, we will have to mention all sorts of topics that can serve only as therapeutic ideals and cannot necessarily be fully implemented. Nevertheless, if we have an overview of what should be considered in treating patients, the details we discover about an illness will yield something of use to us, and at least we will know how to evaluate the inevitably fragmentary conclusions.

Above all, we need to examine the importance of understanding the whole person before us, even when treating the most specialized case. Also this understanding of the human being as a whole should always include the most important events of the patient's life. Members of the medical professions sometimes confide in me and discuss some aspect of a case. After listening to a few words, I have often asked how old the patient was and been astonished to find that the medical professional was unaware of the patient's age and unable to give me any precise information. As we will see in the next few days, it is most important to inform yourself about the patient's age with some degree of accuracy, because therapy is dependent on the age of the patient to a great extent. The day before yesterday, certain therapies were presented as having been extremely helpful in some cases but not in others. In view of such statements, we have to examine the connection between this inefficacy and the age of the patient in question. It is essential to record all the details with regard to how the age of the patient influences the working of therapeutic substances.

Moving on, it is essential to observe carefully how your patient's body has developed. Is this person short and compact, or tall and lanky? The answer is significant because it tells us about the forces of that person's etheric body, as we call it. (I have given this a great deal of thought and have concluded that the use of such terms as etheric body and so forth, which are simply part and parcel of the reality of the human being, is unavoidable, and you would probably not want me to avoid them. We could substitute ones that are more popular among non-anthroposophists, and we may be able to do this at the end of our discussion. But for now, for the sake of better understanding, we will continue to use such terms when necessary.)

The intensity of the working of the etheric body, then, can be assessed on the basis of your patient's growth patterns. As I said, it is not always possible to take everything into account because the information may simply be unavailable, but it is good to know about all this. Whenever possible, it is especially important to enquire about whether the person in question grew quickly or slowly during adolescence. Did he or she remain small for a long time or have a growth spurt at a relatively early age and lag behind later? All of these questions point to what we might call the behaviour of the etheric body, the functional manifestations of the individual in relationship to the physical body, which must be taken into account when we hope to recognize a connection between the patient and particular remedies.

In addition, we must also understand the relationship of the physical and etheric bodies to the higher members of the human constitution, to what we call the astral body (the soul element) and the ego or 'I' (the spiritual element). We need to learn this from our patients. We should not hesitate to ask, for example, whether they dream a lot or only a little. Frequent dreaming is extremely significant for a patient's entire constitution because it shows that the astral body and the ego have a tendency to develop activity of their own and therefore do not want to become involved with the physical body too strongly or in too much detail. As a result, the formative forces of the human soul do not flow into that person's organ systems. Furthermore, even if we are uncomfortable in asking this question, we should also enquire whether the person is active and hard-working or tends to be sluggish. In a personality with a sluggish tendency, the inner mobility of the astral body and the ego is strong. This may sound paradoxical, but this type of mobility does not become conscious; it remains unconscious. And because it is unconscious, the person is not hard-working, even with regard to consciousness, but is sluggish overall. This is because what I call the opposite of sluggishness is the individual's organic capacity for using the higher members to intervene in the lower human being — that is, for leading activity over into the physical and etheric bodies from the astral body and the ego. This capacity is very limited in a sluggish person. From the perspective of spiritual science, a sluggish person is a sleeping person.

After that, we should find out whether our patient is nearsighted or longsighted. A nearsighted person is somewhat reserved with regard to how the ego and astral body relate to the physical body. Nearsightedness is one of the most important signs that you are dealing with a person whose spirit and soul are reluctant to intervene in the physical body.

The next indication is extremely important in treating patients and may become practicable someday. I believe it could acquire practical significance once the individual professions have developed a better sense of cooperation. It is extremely important for dentists to take advantage of everything they know about the teeth, the digestive system, and so on by providing each patient with some sort of checklist after each visit, noting their findings with regard to the development of the patient's teeth, whether there was an early tendency to dental caries, whether the teeth remained in good condition until a later age, and the like. As we will see in the next few days, the condition of the teeth is extremely significant for assessing a person's overall constitution. Making this characteristic signature of the patient's state of health available to the attending physician in the form of a report of dental findings could provide a very significant clue. Of course the patients in question would have to give their consent, but in an atmosphere of cooperation this should be possible.

Next it is extremely important to become aware of the patient's physical likes and dislikes. It is especially significant to determine whether the person you are treating has a craving for salt, for example, or anything else. You would have to find out what foods the person in question craves. If your patient has a particular craving for salty foods, you are dealing with someone with an overly strong connection of the 'I' and the astral body to the physical and etheric bodies. In this person, the spirit and soul have too strong an affinity for the physical body. Dizzy spells brought on by outer mechanical processes, such as rapid turning motions, are also indicative of a strong affinity of this sort. We should ascertain whether mechanical body movements tend to make the patient dizzy. Additionally, as is fairly generally known, we should always find out about any disturbances in secretion, in the patient's overall glandular functioning. When disturbances in secretion are evident, a disturbance is also always present in the ability of the 'I' and astral body to maintain their grip on the etheric and physical bodies.

I have given you some details about what we would always need to know when we meet a patient. I have highlighted details, but you will see where these subjects are pointing in so far as they relate to the constitution of the body itself. As we continue, we will also discuss the need to learn about lifestyle issues—whether or not it is possible for the patient to breathe good air and so forth. We can consider this further when we discuss individual issues. In this way, you will first gain an insight of sorts into the type of person you have to treat. Only when you have acquired such insight will you be in a position, in any specific instance, to know how a particular remedy should be prepared.

Next I would like to mention in general terms an indication that has emerged from some of the lectures in the past few days, namely, the inner relationship of the human being to the entire non-human outer world. Spiritual science often states—although abstractly, to begin with—that in the course of evolution humankind has discharged the other kingdoms from within itself, and that everything external to human beings therefore bears a certain relationship to their own nature and constitution. In contrast to this abstract formulation of our connection with the natural world, we will repeatedly have to point to very specific associations when it comes to the treatment of organs. Above all, however, the basis of the healing relationship between the human being and non-human external nature must first be clear to us.

You know that there is a great deal of debate on this subject and that methods of healing, which we will also discuss in greater detail as we proceed, are engaged in fierce struggles with each other. One struggle in particular is well known—the struggle between physicians who favour homoeopathy and those who think allopathically. It might interest you to know how spiritual science intervenes in this dispute. For today, I will first speak in general terms about this topic and go into the details later. The way in which spiritual science should intervene in this question is actually rather strange. It becomes apparent to spiritual science that there really are no allopathic doctors because even a substance prescribed as an allopathic medication undergoes a process of potentization[1] *within the organism*, and healing occurs only through this process. Thus, all allopathic physicians find their procedures supported by the body's homoeopathic tendency, which brings about a transformation allopaths neglect, namely, breaking down the cohesion of the remedy's individual particles. Admittedly, it does make a considerable difference whether or not we relieve the organism of this potentization process, for the simple reason that healing processes within the organism are probably connected to the state that remedies gradually achieve through potentization. Initially, however, a remedy confronts the body as a foreign entity, as matter that would otherwise belong to the outer world and has no therapeutic relationship to the body. We subject the organism to a great deal of work and disruption if we burden it with all the forces that come to expression when we administer a medication in the allopathic state. We will speak later specifically about cases where it is impossible to relieve the body of this potentizing function.

You see, homoeopathy is a method of healing that has been learned by listening very carefully to nature, at least to some extent, although fanaticism has also brought about significant disjunctures, as we shall see. The important point, however, is to discover ways of relating specific details about the human being to the non-human environment. We cannot, as I said yesterday in a different context, simply parrot the physicians of antiquity, although it can be useful to immerse ourselves in ancient medical literature if we understand it. Instead, for example, we must use all the methods of modern science to explore this interaction between the human being and the non-human environment. First of all, we must realize that chemical investigations of substances—that is, delving into what individual substances reveal in the laboratory—will not get us very far. I have already pointed out that microscopy—and such chemical investigations are also a form of microscopy—ought to be replaced with macroscopic observation, with what is revealed by observing the cosmos itself.

Today I will present significant principles that will point out correspondences between a form of threefold structure in the non-human world and the threefold human being. In this connection, we must look first at the dissolving process. You see, solubility was a property of special importance in the evolution of our planet earth. What precipitated out as the earth's solid portion can be traced back, to a considerable extent, to a cosmic dissolving process that was overcome and killed off, precipitating the solid parts. It is superficial to think only of the mechanical deposition of sediments and to base geognosy[2] and geology entirely on that process. What was primarily involved in the earth-forming process, in incorporating solid components into the body of the earth, consisted of special instances of crystallizing or precipitating out of solution. We can say that to the extent that the dissolving process is something that happens in outer, non-human nature, it is something that human beings have excluded from themselves. External dissolving processes involve activities that human beings have excluded from themselves. The important point here is to investigate the nature of the connection between these processes in the external, non-human cosmos and inner processes in the human organism.

I mentioned earlier that people tend to crave salt when the connection between the spirit and soul and the physical and etheric bodies is overly strong. This is of fundamental importance. These people want to reverse the process of salt precipitation in their own organism, that is, they want to cancel out this earth-forming process, essentially making salt revert to an earlier stage, before solidification in earth's evolution. It is especially important to look at such phenomena because they allow us to investigate the connections between the human organism and outer, non-human nature, to realize that there is an organic need in the nature of the human being to reverse or oppose certain activities that take place in the outer world. As you know, I mentioned yesterday that we even struggle against gravity through development of the buoyancy that supports the human brain. In general, human beings have a tendency to oppose the forces of nature.

[. . .] As we already saw yesterday from other perspectives, the plant represents the opposite of the activity present within the human organism. In the plant itself, however, we can clearly distinguish three different elements. This triple distinction is especially obvious if you look, on the one hand, at everything that delves earthwards in the form of roots, and then at everything that shoots upwards into seeds, fruits and flowers. The contrast between the plant and the human being — although not between the plant and the animal, in this case — is visible even in their external alignment. This contrast is extremely important and significant. The plant sinks into the earth with its roots and pushes upwards with its flowers — that is, with its reproductive organs. With regard to our own orientation in the cosmos, we human beings are the exact opposite. In complete contrast to plants, we 'root' upwards with our heads and push downwards with our reproductive organs. It really makes sense to picture a plant within the human being, a plant that roots upwards and develops its blossom below, in the direction of the reproductive organs. In this way, a particular form of the plant element is incorporated into the human being. Once again, this is an important characteristic for distinguishing between human beings and animals. In an animal, the plant is generally incorporated horizontally, at a right angle to the plant's own direction, while the human being's orientation in the cosmos constitutes a complete 180-degree turn in comparison to the plant.

This is one of the most instructive lessons we can learn by considering the relationship of the human being to the external world. If our medical students would pay more attention to these *macroscopic* findings, they would also discover more about the forces at work in cells, for example, than they would through microscopy. There is actually very little to be gained from microscopy, because the most important forces that are at work in cells can also be observed on the macroscopic level, with variations depending on whether the being in question is a plant, an animal or a human. We can study human cells much better by investigating the interactions among the forces that work vertically upwards, those that work vertically downwards, and those that hold the balance horizontally. These forces which can be observed in the macrocosm work right down into the cellular level. And what is active in cells is essentially nothing other than a copy of this macrocosmic activity.

In studying the earth's plant kingdom, it is critically important to avoid looking at it in the usual manner — that is, by walking around and looking at one plant next to the other, observing the subtle distinctions between them, and inventing a name with two or three parts to establish each plant's place in taxonomy. Instead, you must consider the entire earth as a single being and the whole plant kingdom as belonging to the organism of the earth in the same way that the hairs on your head belong to your own organism (although admittedly your individual hairs are all alike, at least in some respects, while plants differ from each other). An individual plant should no more be considered in isolation than a single hair can be considered an independent organism. That plants differ is due only to the fact that the earth, in its interaction with the rest of the cosmos, develops forces in many different directions. For this reason, plants are structured in different ways, but the life and growth of all plants are based on a single unity within the organization of the earth [...]

[Some] plants tend more towards root formation, devoting a greater proportion of their growth primarily to the roots while the flowers remain small or atrophied. Such plants are more inclined towards earthly factors. In contrast, plants that emancipate themselves from these earthly factors are ones that emphasize the formation of seeds and flowers, and especially those that assume the role of parasites within the plant kingdom. But every plant has a tendency to promote one of its organs to prominence. Just look at how the pineapple plant emphasizes its stem, for example. Or take any other plant. You can say that each of the main plant organs — root, stem, leaf, flower, fruit — becomes the primary organ in some form of plant. Take plants like *Equisetum*, for example. All of their efforts are subsumed in stem formation. Other plants emphasize leaf development, while still others concentrate on flower growth and allow their stems and leaves to atrophy [...]

Everything in the plant that brings about a balance between the flowering and fruiting element and the root element, that is, everything that comes to expression in the leafy parts of ordinary herbaceous plants, will prove to be especially important, even in extract form, for everything that relates to circulatory disturbance—that is, for the rhythmical balance between the upper and lower areas of the body. Earlier in this lecture, we looked at the minerals that internalize intangibles, the minerals that ward off intangibles, and the intermediate types. As you can see now, we find parallels in the overall configuration of the plant. Here you have the very first rational means of establishing an interaction between the human organism and the plant itself, based on the emphasis the plant itself places on developing one or the other of its organs. Later on, we will consider specific manifestations of this interaction [...]

10. Anthroposophical Medicine in Practice: Overview and Three Case Histories

In this final chapter we first summarize some of Steiner's key ideas as we have met them in previous pages, and then, in three case histories – recalling that Steiner refers to his concepts as the necessary but initially empty and abstract cupboard that needs to be fleshed out and filled with life – we see how he put his ideas into practice in the treatment of patients.

Ego and ego organization

In the 'Bridge' lecture (chapter 5), we saw how warm enthusiasm of the ego for moral ideals worked downwards in a conducive way into the other supersensible bodies. The initial aspect of this process is conscious, but as it works down into the body it becomes unconscious.

Then, in chapter 6, various aspects of the ego are mentioned. The part related to sense perception is only tenuously connected to the physical body, but very conscious, while the part that is deeply connected with and 'embodied' in the physical body in movement is unconscious.

The 'Invisible Human Being' lecture (chapter 7) spoke of two aspects of the ego: the conscious, 'naked', direct working of the ego, which has a catabolic or destructive tendency in contrast to the more hidden part that is clothed by the supersensible bodies to work in the blood in an anabolic or synthesizing fashion. This aspect is also mentioned in the lecture on the temperaments (chapter 4) in connection with the constitution of the choleric person.

Inflammation and fever

We saw in the lecture on cancer (chapter 8) that the precondition for inflammation was the etheric body becoming 'slack in one system of organs'. For healing it is necessary to stimulate the etheric organization as a whole. It was also mentioned that inflammation is the opposite of cancer. In chapter 7 Steiner says:

> ... as soon as too much activity is developed in relation to the nerve-sense organization, in a centripetal direction—i.e., when too many outer environment-type processes are 'stuffed' into the human being so that these tumour-like formations develop somewhere, which then fall to pieces—in that moment the other system, which runs along the blood vessels, becomes rebellious. It wants to bring about healing, wants to penetrate the organism with the proper astral and etheric forces that can come from below.

This reactive impulse produces inflammation as a healing effect from 'invisible human being' forces that drive out foreign influences, reasserting the identity of the organism and bringing the body under the individual's control again.

There is evidence that childhood fevers and feverish illness generally act as a protection against cancer developing at a later stage. It is therefore good to let a fever run its course if possible, rather than artificially inhibiting it – though obviously it can be dangerous if it gets out of hand. Doctors and parents frequently notice that children have made progress of some kind after a typical childhood illness, that they have taken a stronger grasp of themselves as individuals. In this sense fever can be a help to the ego in integrating more strongly with the body.

The following two excerpts suggest that in inflammation the astral and ego organization are working too strongly in the metabolic-limb system.

Now let's assume that the digestive organs are too strongly pervaded by the astral body and 'I'. These two members are the active agents driving the digestive portion of the metabolic-limb system. When they work too strongly and become too deeply entrenched, too much digestive activity occurs too quickly. Excessively fast digestion is also incomplete, resulting in diarrhoea and related symptoms.

These symptoms are also associated with another phenomenon, an excess of metabolic-limb activity. Everything works together in the human organism, and excessive metabolic-limb activity works too strongly on both the rhythmic system and the head, especially on the former, where digestive activity continues as digested food is transformed into blood. The rhythm in the blood, in turn, depends on substances entering the blood. When the astral body and 'I' work too strongly, we see symptoms such as fever. Once we know that we can drive the astral body and 'I'-being out of the metabolic-limb system by administering a dose of silver, we also know that silver or its compounds can be used as remedies when the astral body and 'I' are too deeply entrenched in the metabolic-limb system [...]

Now it may also happen that the etheric organism gets the upper hand over the astral, which withdraws. Then there will be rampant growth, which is illness in the other direction. When the astral body gets the upper hand, inflammatory conditions arise; when the etheric activity gets the upper hand, swellings or growths appear. In the entirely normal life of feeling, a delicately poised balance is always maintained between growths and the inflammatory process. The normal life of man needs this possibility of becoming ill, but a continual balancing must take place.

Case histories

Having refreshed for ourselves these concepts of ego, astral, etheric and physical, and their complex dynamic, we will now look at three case histories of patients seen by Steiner and his medical colleague Ita Wegman. A theme running through all these cases is that there are strengthening forces working from the ego organization into the astral which in turn work into the etheric and finally into the physical. As long as this flow takes place in a harmonious way, health is maintained. If it interrupted at any level, various types of illness result.

Case 1

This was a woman aged 26. The whole person showed an extraordinary degree of instability. The patient showed quite clearly that the part of her organism which we have called the astral body in this book was in a state of excessive activity. One saw that this astral body could not be adequately controlled by the ego organization. If the patient wanted to do some work, the astral body immediately came to a boil. The ego organization tried to make itself felt but was constantly repulsed. As a result the temperature goes up in such a case. In a healthy individual, regular digestive activity depends on the ego organization functioning normally. Impotence of this ego organization came to expression as persistent constipation in the patient. A consequence of this problem in the digestive system were the migraine-type conditions and vomiting she presented with. In sleep it is evident that the impotent ego organization causes the organic activity that goes from below upwards to be inadequate, damaging exhalation. The result of this is excessive accumulation of carbon dioxide in the organism during sleep, which shows itself at the organic level as palpitations on waking, and at the psychological level in feelings of anxiety and shouting.

Physical examination showed nothing but a deficit of the forces that bring about a regular relationship between astral body, etheric body and physical body.

Excessive autonomous astral activity means that too few forces flow from the astral body to the physical and etheric body. The latter therefore continue to be delicate in development during the growth period. On examination this was evident from the fact that the patient had a gracefully slender, weak body and complained of frequent back pain. Back pain develops because spinal marrow activity is exactly the site where the ego organization must make itself felt most strongly. The patient also spoke of many dreams. This was due to the astral body evolving excessive independent activity when separated from the physical and etheric body during sleep. As a first step, we had to strengthen the ego organization and reduce astral activity. The first is achieved by selecting a medicine able to support the ego organization where it is getting weak in the digestive tract. Copper may be recognized to be such a medicine. Used in the form of a copper ointment dressing placed over the lumbar region, copper has a strengthening effect on inadequate warmth development which comes from the ego organization. We shall see that abnormal cardiac activity is reduced and the feelings of anxiety disappear. Excessive independent activity of the astral body can be combated with minimal doses of lead taken by mouth.[1] Lead pulls the astral body together and wakes the forces in it through which it combines more strongly with the physical body and the etheric body. (Lead poisoning consists in the astral body being too strongly connected with the etheric body and physical body, so that the latter are subject to an excessive process of destruction.)

The patient showed distinct improvement with this treatment. Her instability gave way to a certain inner firmness and certainty. Her state of mind changed from being fragmented to being inwardly contented. The symptoms of constipation and back pain disappeared, and so did the migraine-like conditions and headaches. The patient regained her ability to work.

Editor's comments on case 1

Constipation
We see in this case history that bowel action is a function of the ego organization. When this withdraws, constipation results.

Migraine
In the 'Constellation' lecture (chapter 6) we saw that in migraine the supersensible bodies in the head behave in the way that they do in the metabolic region, i.e., there is too much metabolic activity in the head.

Nocturnal anxiety and screaming
Inbreathing is a function of the astral and outbreathing a function of the etheric. As the etheric is weakened it is unable to rid

the body of accumulating carbon dioxide, causing anxiety and screaming.

Slight body build
As described in the previous chapter, body build depends on the supersensible bodies working into each other in an anabolic, synthesizing way in early life. When this does not occur properly then slight body build results.

Dreams
As described earlier in the book, having many dreams means that the ego and astral unfold their activity on their own, and are therefore less integrated with the physical.

Case 2

Male patient aged 48; had been robust as a boy, psychologically sound. Stated that he was treated for nephritis for five months during the war and discharged fit. Married at age 35, five healthy children, a sixth died at birth. At age 33, mental over-exertion was followed by depression, tiredness, apathy. These continued to get worse. Parallel to this he felt he had lost his bearings. He faced questions that revealed the negative sides of his work to him—he was a teacher—and he had nothing positive to set against this. The pathological condition showed an astral body with too little affinity to the etheric and physical bodies, and immobile in itself. Because of this, the physical and etheric bodies brought their own inherent qualities into play. The inner feeling of not being properly connected with the astral body caused depression; not being properly connected with the physical body caused tiredness and apathy. The way that the patient felt lost in spirit was due to the fact that the astral body was unable to utilize the physical and etheric body. In connection with all this, sleep was a relief because the astral body had little connection with the etheric and physical body. For the same reason, however, waking up was difficult. The astral body did not want to enter into the physical. A normal connection with the physical and etheric body would only arise in the evening, when they were tired. The patient therefore only really came awake in the evenings. The whole situation indicated that one had first of all to strengthen astral body activity. This can always be achieved by giving a high dilution of arsenic by mouth in form of a natural mineral water.[2] You will find that after some time the individual has more control of his body. The connection between astral body and etheric body grows stronger, depression, apathy and tiredness come to an end. Now it was also necessary to assist the physical body, which had grown sluggish in terms of movement because its connection with the astral body had been poor for a prolonged period, by giving phosphorus in minimal doses. Phosphorus supports the ego organization, enabling it to overcome the resistance of the physical body. Rosemary baths open up a channel for the removal of deposited metabolic products. Eurythmy[3] therapy will restore harmony between the different parts (system of nerves and senses, rhythmic system, motor and metabolic system) of the human organism when it has been upset by inactivity on the part of the astral body. If the patient is also given elderflower tea, the sluggish metabolism which has gradually developed because of inactivity on the part of the astral body will return to normal. We recorded a complete cure in the case of this patient.

Editor's comments on case 2

Depression
We have seen that the etheric body is related to the plant king-
dom. The sun can be understood as a sort of astral force for the
plant. When the sun shines, plants flourish. Similarly, when the
astral works harmoniously into the etheric we feel well and
happy. When this is not the case we become prone to depression.
It is interesting to reflect on the two opposites to the world of
light, i.e., darkness and heaviness, which are both attributes of
depression.

Case 3

A child[4] who had been brought to the clinic twice, first at age 4, then at $5\frac{1}{2}$. Also his mother and the mother's sister. The process of diagnosis led from the child's illness to the mother's and also that of her sister. With the child we found the following. He was a twin, born six weeks prematurely. The other child had died in the final embryonic stage. At the age of six weeks the child fell ill, crying a great deal, and was taken to hospital. Pyloro-spasm was diagnosed. The child was fed partly by a wet nurse, partly artificially. He was discharged from hospital at eight months. On arrival home he had a seizure the first day, and this recurred daily for the first two months. The child would stiffen in an attack, turning up his eyes. Attacks were preceded by timidity and crying. The child also had a squint in the right eye and would vomit before an attack. At age $2\frac{1}{2}$ another attack occurred, lasting five hours. The child went stiff again and lay there as if dead. At age 4 he had an attack lasting 30 minutes. This was the first attack reportedly accompanied by pyrexia. The parents noted that the convulsions that happened after the child came back from hospital were followed by paralysis of the right arm and leg. The child made his first attempts at walking at age $2\frac{1}{2}$. He was only able to step out with the left leg, dragging the right leg after it. The right arm also remained unresponsive to will impulses. The condition still persisted when the child was brought to see us. What we had to do was establish the situation affecting aspects of the child's organization. This was done independently of the syndrome. We found the etheric body to be greatly atrophied, in some parts only accepting a very low level of astral body influence. The region of the right chest was as if paralysed in the etheric body. On the other hand we noted something like a hypertrophy of the astral body in the stomach region. Then the syndrome had to be considered in relation to this. The astral body was clearly putting a considerable strain on the stomach in the digestive process, which, however, was static at the transition from intestine to lymph vessels because of paralysis of the etheric body. This resulted in malnutrition of the blood. The symptoms of nausea and retching thus had to be taken very seriously. Seizures always result if the etheric body grows atrophied and the astral body comes to have a direct influence on the physical body, without mediation from the etheric body. This applied very much in the case of this child. If the condition becomes chronic during the growth period, which was the case here, processes that prepare the motor system to receive the will in the normal way do not occur. This took the form of the child not being able to use the right side.

We then had to connect the child's condition with that of the mother. She was 37 years of age when she came to us. She stated that by the age of 13 she had been as tall as she was now. Her teeth were bad at an early age, she had rheumatic fever as a child and maintained that she had had rickets. Menarche was relatively early. The patient said she had a kidney disease at age 16, and also referred to some kind of seizures she had had. At age 25 she had chronic constipation because of spasms in the anal sphincter, which had to be stretched. She still had spasms with every stool. Diagnosis of her condition, based on direct observation, with no conclusions drawn from her symptom complex, showed remarkable similarity with that of the child, except that everything was much milder in form. It had to be considered that the human etheric body develops especially between the change of teeth and puberty. In the patient this was evident from the fact that the available forces of the etheric body, which were not very strong, made growth possible only until she reached puberty. This is the point where the special development of the astral body began which, being hypertrophic, overwhelmed the etheric body and intervened too strongly in the physical organization. This came to expression in cessation of growth at age 13. The patient was anything but dwarf size, however, and in fact very tall, which was due to the fact that the etheric body's growth forces, uninhibited by the astral body, caused a tremendous increase in the volume of her physical body. These forces were not yet able at the time to intervene in the functions of the physical body in a regular way. This was evident in the development of rheumatic fever and later on of seizures. Because of weakness of the etheric body, the action of the astral body on the physical body was particularly powerful. This was a destructive effect. In normal development it is balanced out by constructive, anabolic forces during sleep, when the astral body has separated from the physical and etheric body. If the etheric body is too weak, as in the case of our patient, excessive catabolic breakdown occurs, and in her case this could be seen from the fact that she needed the first filling in her teeth in her twelfth year. If the etheric body has extra demands made on it, as in pregnancy, this will always cause dental deterioration. The weakness of the etheric body as far as its connection with the astral body was concerned was also particularly evident in the frequency of dreams and in the fact that the patient slept soundly, despite all these irregularities. The weakness of the etheric body was also apparent from the fact that alien processes not controlled by the etheric body occurred in the physical body, presenting as proteins, occasional hyaline casts and salts in her urine.

It is interesting to note the way these pathological processes relate to those of the mother's sister. The diagnosis is almost entirely the same. Weak etheric body activity, therefore dominance of the astral body. In her case, however, the astral body itself is weaker than her sister's. Menarche was therefore early, too, but instead of inflammations she merely had pain due to irritation of the organs, e.g. the joints. The etheric body has to be especially active in the joints if vitality is to develop normally. If etheric body activity is weak the activity of the physical body becomes dominant, which showed in swellings and chronic arthritis in this case. The weakness of the astral body, which is not acting sufficiently on subjective feelings, is evident from a preference for sweet foods, which increase sensation for the astral body. If in addition daily life has worn out a weak astral body, the pain will be more marked if the weakness persists. The patient complained of pain getting worse in the evenings. The connection between the disease states of the three patients pointed to the generation antecedent to the two sisters, and especially the child's grandmother. The cause must lie with her. The upset balance between astral and etheric body in all three patients can only have arisen from an equal imbalance in the child's grandmother. This irregularity must go back to the grandmother's astral and etheric body not achieving adequate nutrition of the foetal membranes which feed the embryo, especially the allantois. This inadequate development of the allantois has to be looked for in all three patients. We established it first of all by purely spiritual methods. The physical allantois is metamorphosed, becoming non-physical, into the capacity of the astral body's forces. A degenerate allantois results in reduced capacity of the astral body, which shows itself especially in all motor organs. All this held true for all three patients. It is indeed possible to perceive the quality of the allantois by considering that of the astral body. It will be evident from this that our reference to a previous generation does not derive from hazardous conclusions based on fantasy but from genuine observations using the methods developed through the science of the spirit. [...]

The mystical concepts of heredity will remain for ever obscure if we shy away from accepting the idea of metamorphosis from physical to non-physical and vice versa in the sequence of generations. As regards treatment, an insight like the above must inevitably give us an idea as to where the healing process should be initiated. If we had not been pointed in the direction of the hereditary aspect but had merely noted the irregularity in the relationship between etheric body and astral body, we would have used medicines that act on these two aspects of the human being. In the present case this would have proved ineffective, however, for the damage, passing through generations, lies too deep to be balanced out in these aspects of the human organization themselves. In a case like this we have to influence the ego organization, bringing everything into play that has to do with harmonizing and strengthening of the etheric body and astral body. We achieve this by addressing the ego organization in enhanced sensory stimuli, as it were (sensory stimuli act on the ego organization). We attempted to do this in the following way for the child. A 5% pyrites ointment dressing was applied to the right hand and at the same time golden agaric ointment (*Amanita caesarea*) was massaged into the left half of the head. Externally applied, pyrites — an iron sulphide — stimulates the ego organization to make the astral body more lively and increase its affinity to the etheric body. The action of golden agaric substance, with organic nitrogen a special constituent, is to let an action going via the ego organization evolve from the head, which makes the etheric body more lively and increases its affinity to the astral body. The healing process was supported by eurythmy therapy, which makes the ego organization as such more lively and active. This results in externally applied principles being taken to the depths of the organization. The healing process thus initiated was further enhanced by measures designed to make astral and etheric body particularly sensitive to the influence of the ego organization. Using a rhythmic diurnal sequence, baths were given with a decoction of *Solidago*, back rubs with a decoction of *Stellaria media*, and both a tea made of willow bark (acts specifically on the astral body's receptivity) and Stannum 0.001 (specifically makes the etheric body receptive) by mouth. We also gave poppy juice in weak homoeopathic doses, to induce the individual's inherently damaged organization to allow the medicinal actions to take effect.

The mother had more of the last of the above treatments, since she was one generation earlier, so that hereditary forces were less involved. The same applied to the mother's sister. We were able to note that while still at the clinic the child was more biddable and the general psychological condition improved. He was more obedient, for instance, and movements that had been very clumsy were done in a more skilful way. Later the aunt reported that the child had gone through a big change. He had become quieter, the excess of involuntary movements was reduced. He has gained sufficient skills to be able to play on his own; and as far as psychological aspects are concerned, his former obstinacy had disappeared.

A passage from chapter 2 of the same book sheds light on the nature of paralysis:

However, thinking also has its physical basis in the organism. It is only that in health it is even more detached from the organism than feeling is. Spiritual perception finds that in addition to the astral body there is a separate ego organization, which lives as an independent soul quality in our thinking. If the human being enters intensely into the bodily aspect with this ego organization, a condition arises in which observation of one's own organism is similar to that of the outside world. If we observe an object or event in the outside world, the fact is that the thought in the human mind and the object or event observed are not in live interaction but independent of each other. This only happens with a human limb if it becomes paralysed. It then becomes 'outside world'. The ego organization is no longer loosely connected with the limb the way it is in health, when it can connect with the limb in a movement and immediately let go again; instead it enters permanently into the limb and can no longer withdraw.

Editor's comments on case 3

Cramps

In the original text it says that cramps (not convulsions) occur when the etheric becomes atrophied and the astral gains a direct influence over the physical without mediation of the etheric body. One is here reminded of the naked ego force working destructively in the nervous system (see chapter 7). Here the flow of anabolic forces from the astral into the etheric has been very weak. This has caused the etheric to atrophy, preventing its mediating action into the physical. The more conscious astral as a consequence works destructively and directly on the physical, causing cramps which manifest as pyloric stenosis as well as epileptic fits.

Paralysis
This is a similar situation for the astral. The ego in the nervous system works in a direct way, directly uniting with the limbs from which it cannot then withdraw.

Growth
We have seen various descriptions of growth in the previous chapter and in chapter 7. Here is yet another aspect. Because the astral does not work strongly into the etheric, growth occurs largely up to puberty only – when the astral body is 'born' or liberated, which then completely inhibits growth.

Constipation
The spasm caused by the direct action of the astral prevents the ego from functioning properly at this level.

Rheumatic fever
In the cancer lecture (chapter 8) we saw how inflammation can be the result of a weak etheric.

Teeth
In the previous chapter we saw how caries is a result of the astral working destructively.

Dreams
We have seen on several occasions that a vivid dream life

indicates a certain independence of the ego and astral, and their lack of connection with the physical.

Conclusion

This book presents something of the wealth of Steiner's insights relating to health and illness. Living and wrestling with them helps us to come to insights ourselves. It will have become clear that these insights are obtained through a means of cognition very different from that underlying natural science. Steiner says that without intuition one cannot really practise medicine.

Though one will not be immediately able to gain such deep, intuitive insights oneself, Steiner shows a very reliable path to tread, which has the same objectivity as science but leads to knowledge of non-physical phenomena and their interaction with the physical.

In medicine based on spiritual science one needs to establish a diagnosis through an intuitive approach, and to experience the interactions of the supersensible bodies. This experience can give rise to a therapeutic impulse, to understanding of which remedies and therapies are appropriate in any instance. The medicines and therapies of course also need to have been transformed into 'experience pictures' too, so that the clinical picture finds its right therapeutic response.

This approach leads to healing on a much deeper, holistic level than is possible in a medicine based on reductionist science.

In the last year of his life, Steiner also gave two lecture cycles which included the use of meditation as a path to deepen

*medicine. The following passage, which concludes this book, is an
excerpt from one of those lectures:*

The forces that enable us to look at things from outside
give us our clear concepts, seeing to it that these clear
concepts do not at once become abstraction but that our
heart thinks with them. Our concepts must not be confused, but the heart must not be excluded from our
abstract thinking. We must function as whole human
beings; the heart must always think as well. We must not
merely think abstractly about the world but realize that
when we send out our thoughts the heart must be there
too. We must understand these forces of the heart which
entwine themselves around thoughts; we must understand once more how to use the staff of Mercury.

Notes

Introduction

1 *Pastoral Medicine: The Collegial Working of Doctors and Priest* (GA 318), Anthroposophic Press, Hudson, NY, 1987.

2 The poisonous spider referred to is *Arania diadema*.

3 *Introducing Anthroposophical Medicine* (GA 312), Anthroposophic Press, 1999.

4 C. Lindenau, *Der Übende Mensch*, Verlag Freies Geistesleben, 1981.

5 Rudolf Steiner 'The Ego as Experience of Consciousness', typescript, available from Rudolf Steiner House Library, London.

Chapter 1

1 Rudolf Steiner and Ita Wegman, *Extending Practical Medicine*, Rudolf Steiner Press, 2000.

2 Very simply put, the etheric body is our 'life' body, related to growth and everything plantlike in us, while the astral body, which we share with the animals, is closely related to soul and emotion. The ego or 'I' is the only aspect of ourselves that is unique and distinct from all other natural kingdoms. Steiner makes these terms clearer in this first chapter.

3 'Natural science' (or 'modern science'), which nowadays is generally referred to just as 'science', is here given its original name by the translator to avoid confusion with 'spiritual science' or 'the science of the spirit'.

4 Imagination in Steiner's terminology (like Intuition and

Inspiration) is usually given a capital 'I' to distinguish it from the more common use of this word.

5 We can thus understand that having developed the faculty Steiner refers to as Imagination, which in his terms is a *tool to perceive reality* rather than an escape from it, we are able to experience the etheric body as an entity distinct from the physical, though also interpenetrating it. Without having developed this faculty of Imagination, however, one can still appreciate the qualities of the etheric by noting the difference the plant demonstrates compared to the mineral, i.e., the plant grows usually in an upward direction towards the light while the roots grow downwards into the earth. It is alive, is usually *green* and has a much more complex morphology etc.

   By converting these attributes into experience one can get an inkling of the nature of the etheric. This Goethean experiential approach is elaborated in the next chapter.

6 This is explained further in the books referred to earlier in the chapter and listed in Further Reading: *How To Know Higher Worlds*, and *Occult Science*.

7 'Astral' comes from the Latin 'astra' meaning 'star'.

8 To appreciate the nature of the astral without developing the higher faculty of Inspiration which Steiner refers to, it is helpful to note the attributes of the animal kingdom. What distinguishes it from the plant kingdom is emotion and movement, and a quite different morphology. The qualitative difference between plant and animal kingdoms is something we can experience by activating our imaginative powers.

9 To appreciate the nature of ego or 'I' without having developed the powers of Intuition that Steiner refers to, it is helpful to enumerate the attributes that differentiate the

human from the animal, e.g. upright posture, speech, thinking, morality and freedom of action. Again, these need to be imaginatively experienced in order to experience the qualitative difference between man and animal.

10   In other words, the astral and 'I' principles are what inform and imbue the physical and etheric bodies in order for us to live as human beings.

Chapter 2

1   In German, *anschauende Urteilskraft*. Very loosely translated, this means the power of intuitive judgement drawing on creative perception.

2   In other words, experiences are precognitive: we have them before thinking arises out of them.

Chapter 3

1   See chapter 1, note 2, and also chapter 4.

2   The consciousness soul is Steiner's term for wide-awake, self-aware consciousness, and the capacity to take responsibility for one's actions. Inherent in it is a sense of being separate from the world, standing alone as an individual.

3   By 'ego' Steiner does not mean the 'lower ego' we normally understand by this term, which is capable of 'egotism', but a much higher principle — the essential innate core of an individual human being.

4   Two stages in the evolution of human consciousness that precede the consciousness soul. At the sentient soul stage we relate to the world through our impulsive feelings and immediate emotional response. The intellectual or mind soul reflects on the world through thinking but does not yet attain the greater self-awareness of the consciousness soul.

5   The 'Dark Age' during which spiritual vision was clouded and man's attention focused increasingly on the material world alone.

Chapter 4

1   It is a central aspect of Steiner's ideas on reincarnation and karma that the people we meet and events that happen to us are not by pure chance but inwardly dictated by our own innermost and unconscious intentions. Also see note 3 below.

2   The physical, etheric and astral bodies and ego.

3   Reincarnation is a central tenet of Steiner's anthroposophy. The essential individuality sheds the other 'bodies' at death, and dwells in the spiritual world until the urge to reincarnate in a new body becomes sufficiently strong. In this way, according to Steiner, each of us has participated in all evolutionary stages of the earth.

Chapter 5

1   René Descartes, 1596–1650, French philosopher. Cartesian dualism holds that mind is a thinking but non-extended substance which is distinct from any matter that may exist, while matter is an extended and non-thinking substance. (R. L. Arrington, *A Companion to the Philosophers*, Blackwell, Massachusetts, 1999). In other words, mind and matter are two quite separate spheres that represent an unbridgeable divide.

2   L. Le Shan, *You Can Fight For Your Life*, Thorsons, 1984.

3   It would go beyond the scope of this book to try to explain the four ethers which Steiner refers to here. They are four different aspects or qualities that compose the etheric body of formative forces.

4   A law formulated by Julius Robert Mayer (1814–78).

Chapter 6

1   Published in *Anthroposophical Spiritual Science and Medical Therapy*, Mercury Press, NY, 1991.

Chapter 7

1   L. Le Shan, *You Can Fight For Your Life*, Thorsons, London, 1984.

2   For more on stages of evolution as described by Steiner, see *An Outline of Esoteric Science*, Anthroposophic Press, Hudson, NY, 1997.

Chapter 8

1   See R. Leroi, 'Der Ätherleib zwischen Kosmos und Erde. Beitrag zum Verständnis der Karzinomentstehung'. In: *Beitrag zu einer Erweiterung der Heilkunst*, Jan/Feb. 1983.

2   R. Grossarth-Maticek, H. Kiene, S. Baumgartner, R. Ziegler, 'Use of Iscador, an extract of European mistletoe (*Viscum album*), in cancer treatment: prospective non-randomized and randomized matched-pairs studies nested within a cohort study.' Published in the peer-reviewed journal *Alternative Therapies*, May–June 2001.

3   The English equivalent would be 'to do its own thing'.

4   A technique of serial dilution used in homoeopathic medicine. Through progressive series of dilutions very little of the original substance, if any, still remains, but the progress aims to leave an imprint of the substance's essential pattern and dynamic on the fluid in which it is diluted.

5   Steiner is here referring to natural remedies, not, of course, to modern psychotropic drugs.

6   This passage can only be understood if we take the etheric forces as being *foreign* etheric forces behaving as a tissue

culture (see editor's introduction to this chapter, and note 2).

7   The astral body is closely related to the animal kingdom, and the etheric body to the plant kingdom. Steiner is therefore suggesting that we need to find in the natural world a substance that reflects what is insufficiently strong in the human being.

Chapter 9

1   See note 4 on potentizing in chapter 8.
2   The study of the earth, its structure and strata. This includes geology, which studies the earth's crust.

Chapter 10

1   The form of lead used was a homoeopathic potency: Plumbum 10x.
2   Levico water from Italy has a natural arsenic content.
3   Movements based on the sounds of speech and music made visible, and used to harmonize the supersensible bodies.
4   The gender of the child is unknown, but will be referred to here as 'he'.

Sources

The GA [*Gesamtausgabe*] numbers refer to the volume number in the original German edition of Steiner's works.

Chapter 1
Rudolf Steiner and Ita Wegman, *Extending Practical Medicine*, GA 27, Rudolf Steiner Press, 2000, from chapter 1

Chapter 2
The Science of Knowing, GA 2, Mercury Press, 1988, pp. 86–100

Chapter 3
Metamorphosis of the Soul, GA 58, Rudolf Steiner Press, 1983, pp. 54–59
Education for Special Needs, GA 317, Rudolf Steiner Press, 1998, from lecture 10

Chapter 4
The Four Temperaments, GA 57, Rudolf Steiner Publishing Co., 1944, pp. 21–39

Chapter 5
The Bridge Between Universal Spirituality and the Physical Constitution of the Human Being (contained also in the *Course for Young Doctors*), GA 202, Anthroposophic Press, 1958, pp. 7–41

Chapter 6
'Human Becoming World Soul and World Spirit', GA 205, typescript available from Rudolf Steiner House Library, London.

Chapter 7
Earthly Knowledge and Heavenly Wisdom, GA 221, Anthroposophic Press, 1991, pp. 69–86

Chapter 8
Introducing Anthroposophical Medicine, GA 312, Anthroposophic Press, 1999, lecture 12
The Healing Process, GA 319, Anthroposophic Press, 2000, from lecture 10
Fundamentals of Anthroposophical Medicine, GA 218, Mercury Press, 1986, pp. 56–59

Chapter 9
Introducing Anthroposophical Medicine, GA 312, Anthroposophic Press, 1999, from lecture 5

Chapter 10
The Healing Process, GA 319, Anthroposophic Press, 2000, p. 134
Course For Young Doctors, GA 316, Mercury Press, n.d., pp. 18, 186–7
Extending Practical Medicine, GA 27, Rudolf Steiner Press, 2000, chapters 2 and 19

Further reading

Works by Rudolf Steiner

Anthroposophical Spiritual Science and Medical Therapy, Mercury Press, Spring Valley, NY, 1991

Anthroposophy and Science: Observation, Experiment, Mathematics, Mercury Press, Spring Valley, NY, 1991

Bridge Between Universal Spirituality and the Physical Constitution of Man, Anthroposophic Press, Spring Valley, NY, 1958

Extending Practical Medicine: Fundamental Principles Based on the Science of the Spirit (written by Rudolf Steiner & Ita Wegman MD), Rudolf Steiner Press, London, 1996

How to Know Higher Worlds: A Modern Path of Initiation, Anthroposophic Press, Hudson, NY, 1994

Intuitive Thinking as a Spiritual Path: A Philosophy of Freedom, Anthroposophic Press, Hudson, NY, 1995

Karmic Relationships: Esoteric Studies, 8 vols, Rudolf Steiner Press, London, 1974–97.

Nutrition and Stimulants, Bio-Dynamic Farming and Gardening Association, Kimberton, PA, 1991

An Outline of Esoteric Science, Anthroposophic Press, Hudson, NY, 1997 (also published as *Occult Science*)

The Origin of Suffering, The Origin of Evil, Illness, and Death, Steiner Book Centre, North Vancouver, 1980

Pastoral Medicine: The Collegial Working of Doctors and Priests, Anthroposophic Press, Hudson, NY, 1987

Polarities in Health, Illness, and Therapy, Mercury Press, Spring Valley, NY, 1987

Psychoanalysis & Spiritual Psychology. Anthroposophic Press, Hudson, NY, 1990

A Psychology of Body, Soul, & Spirit, introduced by Robert Sardello, Anthroposophic Press, Hudson, NY, 1999 (previous translations were titled *Anthroposophy, Psychosophy, Pneumatosophy* and *The Wisdom of Man, of the Soul, and of the Spirit*)

Therapeutic Insights: Earthly and Cosmic Laws, Mercury Press, Spring Valley, NY, 1984

Theosophy: An Introduction to the Spiritual Processes in Human Life and in the Cosmos, Anthroposophic Press, Hudson, NY, 1994

What Can the Art of Healing Learn through Spiritual Science? Mercury Press, Spring Valley, NY, 1986

Other authors:

Bortoft, Henri, *The Wholeness of Nature: Goethe's Way Toward a Science of Conscious Participation in Nature,* Lindisfarne Books, Hudson, NY, 1996

Emmichoven, F.W. Zeylmans van, *The Anthroposophical Understanding of the Soul,* Anthroposophic Press, Hudson, NY, 1982.

Evans, Dr Michael and Iain Rodger, *Anthroposophical Medicine: Healing for Body, Soul and Spirit*, Thorsons, London, 1992

Hauschka, Margarethe, MD *Rhythmical Massage: As Indicated by Ita Wegman*, MD, Rudolf Steiner Press, London, 1979

Holdrege, Craig, *Genetics and the Manipulation of Life: The Forgotten Fact of Context*, Lindisfarne Books, Hudson, NY, 1996

Holtzapfel, Walter, *The Human Organs: Their Functional and Psychological Significance*, The Lanthorn Press, 1993.

Husemann, Friedrich, & Otto Wolff, eds, *The Anthroposophical Approach to Medicine*, 3 vols, Anthroposophic Press, Hudson, NY, 1989

Lehrs, Ernst, *Man or Matter: Introduction to a Spiritual Understanding of Nature on the Basis of Goethe's Method of Training Observation and Thought*, 3rd edition, Rudolf Steiner Press, London, 1985

Lievegoed, Bernard, *Man on the Threshold*, Hawthorn Press, Stroud, 1985

— *Phases: The Spiritual Rhythms of Adult Life*, Rudolf Steiner Press, 1993

McDermott, Robert A., *The Essential Steiner*, Harper Collins, San Francisco, 1984

Mees, L.C.F., MD, *Blessed By Illness*, Anthroposophic Press, Hudson, NY, 1983

Pearce, Joseph Chilton, *Evolution's End: Claiming the Potential of Our Intelligence*, Harper Collins, NY, 1992

Priever, Werner, MD, *Illness and the Double*, Mercury Press, Spring Valley, NY, 1982

Roszell, Calvert, *The Near-Death Experience*, Anthroposophic Press, Hudson, NY, 1992

Treichler, Rudolf, *Soulways: The Developing Soul-Life Phases, Thresholds and Biography*, Hawthorn Press, Stroud, 1989

Weihs, Thomas, *Embryogenesis in Myth and Science*, Floris Books, Edinburgh, 1986

Acknowledgements

I would like to thank Dr G. Douch who was such a help with corrections, and Frank Mulder who made helpful comments on the text and supplied suggestions. I would also like to thank Matthew Barton for his careful revision.

Note Regarding Rudolf Steiner's Lectures

The lectures and addresses contained in this volume have been translated from the German, which is based on stenographic and other recorded texts that were in most cases never seen or revised by the lecturer. Hence, due to human errors in hearing and transcription, they may contain mistakes and faulty passages. Every effort has been made to ensure that this is not the case. Some of the lectures were given to audiences more familiar with anthroposophy; these are the so-called 'private' or 'members' lectures. Other lectures, like the written works, were intended for the general public. The difference between these, as Rudolf Steiner indicates in his *Autobiography*, is twofold. On the one hand, the members' lectures take for granted a background in and commitment to anthroposophy; in the public lectures this was not the case. At the same time, the members' lectures address the concerns and dilemmas of the members, while the public work speaks directly out of Steiner's own understanding of universal needs. Nevertheless, as Rudolf Steiner stresses: 'Nothing was ever said that was not solely the result of my direct experience of the growing content of anthroposophy. There was never any question of concessions to the prejudices and preferences of the members. Whoever reads these privately printed lectures can take them to represent anthroposophy in the fullest sense. Thus it was possible without hesitation—when the complaints in this direction became too persistent—to depart from the custom of circulating this material "For members only". But it must be borne in mind that faulty passages do occur in these reports not revised by myself.' Earlier in the same chapter, he states: 'Had I been able to correct them [*the private lectures*], the restriction *for members only* would have been unnecessary from the beginning.'

The original German editions on which this text is based were published by Rudolf Steiner Verlag, Dornach, Switzerland in the collected edition (*Gesamtausgabe*, 'GA') of Rudolf Steiner's work. All publications are edited by the Rudolf Steiner Nachlassverwaltung (estate), which wholly owns both Rudolf Steiner Verlag and the Rudolf Steiner Archive. The organization relies solely on donations to continue its activity.

For further information please contact:

Rudolf Steiner Archiv
Postfach 135
CH-4143 Dornach

or:

www.rudolf-steiner.com

ALSO AVAILABLE IN THE 'POCKET LIBRARY OF
SPIRITUAL WISDOM' SERIES:

AGRICULTURE

Compiled with an introduction, commentary and notes by
Richard Thornton Smith

The evolving human being
Cosmos as the source of life
Plants and the living earth
Farms and the realms of nature
Bringing the chemical elements to life
Soil and the world of spirit
Supporting and regulating life processes
Spirits of the elements
Nutrition and vitality
Responsibility for the future

ISBN 1 85584 113 4; £8.95

ARCHITECTURE

Compiled with an introduction, commentary and notes by
Andrew Beard

The origins and nature of architecture
The formative influence of architectural forms
The history of architecture in the light of mankind's spiritual
   evolution
A new architecture as a means of uniting with spiritual forces
Art and architecture as manifestations of spiritual realities
Metamorphosis in architecture
Aspects of a new architecture
Rudolf Steiner on the first Goetheanum building
The second Goetheanum building
The architecture of a community in Dornach
The temple is the human being
The restoration of the lost temple

ISBN 1 85584 123 1; £9.95

ART

Compiled with an introduction, commentary and notes by Anne Stockton

The being of the arts
Goethe as the founder of a new science of aesthetics
Technology and art
At the turn of each new millennium
The task of modern art and architecture
The living walls
The glass windows
Colour on the walls
Form — moving the circle
The seven planetary capitals of the first Goetheanum
The model and the statue 'The Representative of Man'
Colour and faces
Physiognomies

ISBN 1 85584 138 X; £9.95

EDUCATION

Compiled with an introduction, commentary and notes by
Christopher Clouder

A social basis for education
The spirit of the Waldorf school
Educational methods based on anthroposophy
The child at play
Teaching from a foundation of spiritual insight and education in
    the light of spiritual science
The adolescent after the fourteenth year
Science, art, religion and morality
The spiritual grounds of education
The role of caring in education
The roots of education and the kingdom of childhood
Address at a parents' evening
Education in the wider social context

ISBN 1 85584 118 5; £8.95

RELIGION

Compiled with an introduction, commentary and notes by
Andrew Welburn

Mysticism and beyond: the importance of prayer
The meaning of sin and grace
Rediscovering the Bible
What is true communion?
Rediscovering the festivals and the life of the earth
Finding one's destiny: walking with Christ
The significance of religion in life and death
Christ's second coming: the truth for our time
Universal religion: the meaning of love

ISBN 1 85584 128 2; £8.95

SCIENCE

Compiled with an introduction, commentary and notes by
Howard Smith

From pre-science to science
The origin of mathematics
The roots of physics and chemistry, and the urge to experiment
Are there limits to what science can know?
Understanding organisms: Goethe's method
The quest for archetypal phenomena
Light, darkness and colour;
The rediscovery of the elements
What is warmth?
The scale of nature
The working of the ethers in the physical
Sub-nature; What are atoms?
Natural science and spiritual science

ISBN 1 85584 108 8; £8.95

SOCIAL AND POLITICAL SCIENCE

Compiled with an introduction, commentary and notes by
Stephen E. Usher

Psychological cognition
The social question
The social question and theosophy
Memoranda of 1917
The metamorphosis of intelligence
Culture, law and economy
Central Europe between East and West

ISBN 1 85584 103 7; £8.95